BRACING ACCOUNTS

BRACING ACCOUNTS

The Literature and Culture
of Polio in Postwar America

Jacqueline Foertsch

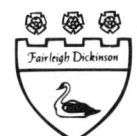

Madison • Teaneck
Fairleigh Dickinson University Press

©2008 by Rosemont Publishing & Printing Corp.

All rights reserved. Authorization to photocopy items for internal or personal use, or the internal or personal use of specific clients, is granted by the copyright owner, provided that a base fee of $10.00, plus eight cents per page, per copy is paid directly to the Copyright Clearance Center, 222 Rosewood Drive, Danvers, Massachusetts 01923. [978-0-8386-4173-6/08 $10.00 + 8¢ pp, pc.]

Associated University Presses
2010 Eastpark Boulevard
Cranbury, NJ 08512

The paper used in this publication meets the requirements of the American National Standard for Permanence of Paper for Printed Library Materials Z39.48–1984.

Library of Congress Cataloging-in-Publication Data

Foertsch, Jacqueline, 1964–
 Bracing accounts : the literature and culture of polio in postwar America / Jacqueline Foertsch.
   p. cm.
 Includes bibliographical references and index.
 ISBN 978-0-8386-4173-6 (alk. paper)
 1. American literature—20th century—History and criticism. 2. Poliomyelitis—Patients—United States—Biography—medicine—United States—History—20th century. I. Title.

PS228.P57F64 2008
810.9'3561—dc22
                        2008014064

PRINTED IN THE UNITED STATES OF AMERICA

Contents

Acknowledgments 7

Introduction. Reality and Its Representations:
Stories from the American Polio Era 11

1. "A Battle of Silence":
Women's Magazines in the Postwar Polio Era 26

2. "No Time for Tears"?:
Gender, Fiction, and Denial in Polio Memoirs 51

3. "Crippled by History":
Polio and the Past in Contemporary Novels 97

4. "Heads, You Win!":
Newsletters and Magazines of the Polio Nation 135

Conclusion. "The Voice is Still There":
Some Final Notes on Postwar Polio Culture 170

Notes 183

Works Cited 209

Index 219

Acknowledgments

THE WRITING OF THIS BOOK WAS FUNDAMENTALLY ASSISTED BY MANY generous groups and individuals: the NEH Summer Stipend program and the University of North Texas's Junior Faculty Summer Research and Faculty Research Grant programs provided invaluable summer support for the completion of various chapters and revisions; Deirdre Clarkin, Rose LaBarge, and their assistants at the National Library of Medicine and staff at the Library of Congress were of great help in my on-site research, as were David Rose, archivist at the March of Dimes Foundation, and Claude B. Zachary and his staff at the University of Southern California's Doheny Memorial Library, where the Rancho Los Amigos collection is housed. My thanks as well to the staff at AFB Research; to J. Archer O'Reilly III, Director of Information and Editor of *Disability Issues*; to Dorothy Nattrass, National Welfare Officer at the British Polio Fellowship; and to Dean Hendrix and Linda Lohr at the University of Buffalo Health Sciences Library. Special thanks to Richard Dagget; Alice Willetts; Susanne Williams, Director of Consumer and Reader Services at *Good Housekeeping*; Joan Headley, editor of the *Rehabilitation Gazette* (for answering all my questions) and to Warm Springs Senior Librarian Michael D. Shadix, whose advice and assistance over many years have been invaluable. Thanks to friend and mentor David Kesterson for thinking of me whenever polio-related material crossed his desk. Thanks also to G. Thomas Couser for his advice and support and to Douglas Field, Ronald Corthell (editor) and the readers at *Prose Studies*, and the editors and readers at *Disability Studies Quarterly*, especially Brenda Brueggemann and Stephen Kuusisto, for their revision suggestions and for their publication of my work. I am grateful as well to the readers, editors, and production staffs at Fairleigh Dickinson University Press and Associated University Presses, especially Harry Keyishian, for their interest in and encouragement of my work.

Finally, my thanks to dear colleagues, friends, and family—for whom I write always. This book is dedicated to darling Aurora and Solana, who are fancy young ladies now.

∽ ∽ ∽

I gratefully acknowledge the print sources where materials adapted for this book have previously appeared: parts of chapter 1 appeared as "A Battle of Silence: Women's Magazines and the Polio Crisis in Post-war UK and USA" in *American Cold War Culture* (ed. Douglas Field, Edinburgh University Press, 2005); parts of chapter 2 appeared as "No Time for Tears?: Gender and Denial in Polio Memoirs" in *Prose Studies* 29, no. 2 (www.informaworld.com); and parts of chapter 4 appeared as "'Heads, You Win!': Newsletters and Magazines of the Polio Nation" in *Disability Studies Quarterly* 27, no. 3.

BRACING ACCOUNTS

Introduction
Reality and Its Representations: Stories from the American Polio Era

It is the middle of the twentieth century and very hot outside. In the midst of a schedule filled with work and family, or school and play, a young protagonist gets a fever and stiff neck and takes to bed, often "never to rise unassisted again." Family members are summoned, a feverish ride to the hospital ensues. Following the perfunctory spinal tap, it is always polio. Parents are banished, and a silence falls; as Robert F. Hall movingly recalls, "a nurse came to the door of my room and closed it. She did so without saying a word. That is how I learned I had polio. I was very much alone."[1]

Intense pain and high fever accompany the onset of longer-term effects: in a spinal case, paralysis creeps up one side and down the other; the patient may sit in bed lucidly observing this phenomenon, wondering when sensation will return or bidding mobility farewell forever. In a bulbar case, when polio attacks motor neurons in the brainstem, the onset of an intensely nasal, stilted speech makes communication difficult, swallowing is hindered by an extreme sore throat, and in the worst cases breathing seizes to a trickle and the patient requires a respirator, the dreaded iron lung. While this is often a temporary stay, or only a treatment applied to the patient in the next bed, the terrors of the respirator resonate throughout the story. Again, Hall: "It was [a fellow-patient's] hissing respirator that whispered to me, 'You're next.'"[2] Despite the protagonist's sometimes dire situation, there is often someone in the next bed or down the hall worse off.

When the fever and sharpest pains subside, rehabilitation begins: steaming wool hot packs (whose distinctive odor lingers in the memory decades later) and daily stretching exercises. These treatments are dispensed by a range of personalities: benign, handsome doctors (who are also usually young and blond), sadistic older nurses (often those on the overnight shift), and inept physical therapists. A radio is donated, connecting the patient to beloved classical music and/or the weekly adventures of serial cowboy Tom Mix. Watching a ballgame on TV in the mirror over his head, the patient-protagonist sees the batter running "backwards" around the bases. Breathing eventually normalizes, and more and more time is spent freed of the iron contraption. Following weeks or months of improvement, the momentous brace/chair intersection is reached: will the patient attain verticality once more? It is always an amazingly "long way down" the first time s/he stands after so many bedridden months. Sometimes a disastrous fall means permanent wheelchair usage and a life-long battle for greater access to public places, while sometimes braces and crutches enable long walks and successful stair-climbing.

Emotional recovery occurs in the formation of friendships with fellow-"polios" (the term of reference in that period, largely discredited today) of both sexes and all ages and ability levels. Holidays are shared, satiric shows presented for family and staff, and the end of the convalescent period, so full of progress, fun, and acceptance by others, is met with trepidation. In the outside world the polio survivor faces condescending sympathy, rude stares, and a disinclination to associate with other disabled people—at least at first—that is fiercely reciprocated. Job finding may be an issue, but marriage usually is not; world travel is embarked upon when the opportunity presents itself, and a frequent career of choice is college professor. At the end of the story, the polio-affected subject looks back on a record of courage and achievement; physical or at least emotional health has been restored, and with rare exception no one dies.

The literary elements in the preceding account—my reference to the polio-affected youngster as a "protagonist," my insistence that by story's end all are alive and well—are meant to indicate the nature of the project commencing here, which departs from the many valuable histories of polio published in the last decade or two, and especially in the very recent past, surrounding the fiftieth anniversary of the Salk vaccine.[3] While vitally informed by these other works, *Bracing Accounts* explores the field of polio's textual representation, interrogating the cultural, ideological, and therapeutic roles played by polio-related journalism, memoirs, novels, and newsletters for those within and those outside the polio experience from the postwar era to the present day. The above account is a composite of numerous diverse polio-themed works, specifically polio memoirs, and rehearses a recurring plotline of the genre, especially from the immediate postwar era. These memoirs, observes Jane Smith,

> resemble the most formulaic of war movies, the kind where a disparate crew is sent on a dangerous mission and, in the process, discovers the true meaning of fellowship. Every polio ward, it seemed, like every Hollywood fighter squadron, contained a wisecracking optimist, a poetic cynic, a hero, a traitor, a brave lad who died and another who made it home for Christmas. Every hospital had a beautiful nurse with soothing hands, a sadistic one who kept the strictest of rules, and a doctor who would arrive to make the rounds and offer hope when morale was at its very lowest.[4]

Such consistent textual patterning indicates the strikingly "universal" experience that was polio illness and recovery, even as it belies the relatively rare occurrence of actual symptomatic infection, as well as the notoriously random and unknowable aspects of the disease when it did occur. For like a medieval wheel of fortune, where polio stopped, no one knew: how it entered the body and moved among populations, whether it would strike this town or that, why summer was such a dangerous season, how extensive or permanent the damage in each case would be, were guessing (or waiting) games played by patients, physicians, and families countless times during the polio period.[5] Decades after what is thought to be successful recovery (and even after an abortive childhood infection that produced no symptoms at the time), post-polio syndrome may threaten an aging body with a range of symptoms and limitations.

While the disease has had many names, "poliomyelitis" was coined in the early twentieth century to describe its inflammatory attack (*itis*) of the gray (*polios*) anterior matter of the spinal cord (*myelos*). During the regrettable decades of constant usage, the term was shortened to "polio"; the earlier term "infantile paralysis" (or even just "infantile") hung on in some quarters, even though its victims were more and more often older children and even young adults. Symptomatic polio onset involved fatigue, headache, and stiff neck; following an acute, infectious phase of high fever and intense pain, the nerves responsible for various muscle movement sustained either damage or destruction, resulting in temporary or permanent contracture, shrinkage, and paralysis. Bulbar and bulbospinal forms of polio affected breathing muscles and required placing the patient inside an iron lung, a metal canister containing everything but the patient's head, which used a rubber gasket fitted snugly around the neck to create an airtight, negative-pressure ventilation system involving bellows and a vacuum effect to move the paralyzed diaphragm up and down. While much has been learned about polio since the early twentieth century—its viral identity, its antigenic typology, its enteric (intestinal) situation in the body, its passing among persons through hand-to-hand or hand-to-mouth fecal residue—"there is much about the disease that remains a mystery. . . . Why was polio among the most seasonal of afflictions, with thirty-five times as many cases in August than in April? What made children so susceptible to the virus, especially boys?"[6] Given polio's many enduring enigmas and the markedly individualized course of illness and debility suffered by each polio patient/survivor, we may begin to discern vital distinctions between the polio experience in its immeasurable variation and the polio *story*—its fictions, revelations, and rhetorical strategies—even as the story frequently succeeds in representing the experience with remarkable poignancy and significance.

In *Bracing Accounts*, I will discuss specific genres of polio literature in the United States, popularized throughout the second half of the twentieth century, as well as the interaction between the individual text and its concession to the market (i.e., ideological) demand that a redemptive story be told. Smith observes that "the very titles of books about polio [e.g., *Rise Up and Walk* and *My Place to Stand*] show the required dose of jaunty uplift."[7] Regarding illness narrative in general, G. Thomas Couser notes that "those with chronic illness or disability" must "reconcil[e] their illness with the comic plot expected of autobiography" or go unpublished.[8] The bestselling account may arc through its crises and resolutions with so insistent an upswing—we should picture not a rainbow but a smile—that it comes full circle. Arthur W. Frank looks suspiciously upon the "restitution narrative," which only concludes when the patient-narrator fully reinhabits his original self, rendering the journey through the illness experience meaningless.[9] His point is well taken and enlarged upon in this book: while I recognize denial as a vital coping strategy in the lived experience of recovering from (or adjusting to) traumatic illness and impairment, I am interested to explore here the text-in-denial as a specific phenomenon, considering the polio narrative's divided allegiance to the authenticity of experience and to publication itself. Meanwhile, I gaze as appreciatively upon aspects of denial in polio texts as I do instances of realistic, complex exploration of the illness, recovery, impairment, and disability experiences surrounding polio. For even the formulaic approach is instructive regarding not only polio illness and recovery but, perhaps even more valuably, the diffidence surrounding death, impairment, depression, and other forms of bad news resulting from serious illness that shaped mass-marketed narratives of illness during the polio era and continue to do so today.

Likely occurrences of polio have been recorded—indeed, etched in stone tablets—since 1500 BC. For centuries it was largely endemic in the human population, causing mild illness then conferring lifetime immunity. Only since the industrial era, when modern sanitation methods separated children from the necessary early exposure and prevented immunities from developing, did the disease shift from isolated incident to regular, even annual event. Throughout the late nineteenth and early twentieth centuries, epidemics were reported with some frequency in Western Europe and the United States; in 1916, the boroughs of New York experienced a major outbreak, after which "there was not a year that passed without an epidemic somewhere."[10] Following hard on the heels of the Depression and the Second World War, the United States in the late 1940s and early 1950s saw record infection rates—the highpoint was 1952 with some 58,000 cases—that abruptly trailed off (as did research interest in the disease as a whole) with the advent of the Salk vaccine in 1955. Following a massive 1954 field trial involving 1.8 million schoolchildren, the vaccine was announced to be safe and effective in March 1955 to thunderous public acclaim. While Salk was dismissed by his fellow scientists for failing to break new ground and for over-actively seeking the limelight, his vaccine changed the life of every American and was the crowning achievement of Franklin Delano Roosevelt's March of Dimes campaign to eradicate the disease.

Roosevelt is the most famous polio-affected person in U.S. history, having contracted the disease in 1921 at the age of thirty-nine, while vacationing with his family on Campobello Island off the coast of New Brunswick, Canada.[11] Following a stressful period involving scandal during his tenure as assistant secretary of the Navy and a hectic day of exercise and fatigue, Roosevelt experienced high fever, pain, and paralysis. He was diagnosed with polio, which would leave him permanently paralyzed in both legs, though he labored mightily to regain movement and hid his impairment from public view much of his life. Having heard about the healthful properties of swimming in warm water springs in the mountains of northern Georgia, Roosevelt purchased an area resort, the Meriwether Inn, and its decrepit environs in 1926 and transformed it into the Georgia Warm Springs Foundation, the nation's leading polio rehabilitation facility. During the Depression, when the curtailment of private donations threatened the Foundation's existence, then-New York Governor Roosevelt turned to his young law partner and Foundation director, Basil O'Connor, to start up a national organization to fund Warm Springs, care for the polio-affected in local communities, and spearhead research. Beginning in 1934, the National Foundation for Infantile Paralysis sponsored hugely popular annual balls on the president's birthday (January 30), whose motto was "We Dance, So that Others May Walk."

When the novelty of these gatherings wore off and another fundraising idea was needed, film star and Roosevelt-devotee Eddie Cantor coined the term "The March of Dimes" in 1938, riffing on the popular "March of Time" newsreel series that opened many a Hollywood feature. Cantor invited his expansive radio audience (largely comprised of children) to send their dimes to the White House; the response was overwhelming, and the nationalizing of the polio problem—and its eventual solution—began. The March of Dimes created an all-media environment—posters, newsreels, star-studded awareness campaigns—as pervasive and persuasive as the one created by the Office of War Information during the early 1940s. The posters featured charming, well-dressed toddlers cosseted in braces or breaking free of these; the rattling collection can, one even tipped sidewise and mounted on legs like a miniature iron lung, was a persistent reminder in film theaters, on street corners, and at school. David Oshinsky helpfully outlines the history of small-gift philanthropy in twentieth-century America, beginning with Liberty Bonds to support the First World War and flourishing throughout the polio decades of the 1940s and 1950s.[12] The March of Dimes eventually collected millions (of dollars and dimes) and sent these proceeds to local chapters to help families with hospital bills and home care, to pay for braces and iron lungs, and to perpetuate an awareness campaign that made polio into a household name and a cause of universal concern. In Oshinsky's striking assessment, "Polio's special status was due, in large part, to . . . the National Foundation . . . , which employed the latest techniques in advertising, fund raising, and motivational research to turn a horrific but relatively uncommon disease into the most feared affliction of its time."

Regardless of the role played specifically by the March of Dimes, for the vast majority of Americans, polio entered the postwar home (and the school and the movie theater) solely as textual representation, not biological event. Even during America's peak polio years (in the late 1940s and early 1950s), few were visibly affected by its infectious and paralyzing processes, even fewer required respirator assistance, and fewer yet died from the disease: its most serious outcomes, however, involving small children hobbling on crutches and braces or succumbing to death in an iron lung, were so pervasively depicted for an ever-increasing parental populace in postwar, baby-boom America that polio became a universal terror. Polio's appearance during summer months, when its youthful targets were at their ostensible freest, forced parents into the dilemma of which would do worse damage—spoiling a child's leisure time year after year (by keeping him from summer camp, the public pool, or movie house, by forcing her indoors for long hours every afternoon) against the low odds of actual infection, or failing to do so.

That polio was far more often a psychological torment than a realized physical problem means that polio-related cultural texts responded to (sprung from, alleviated, exacerbated) national anxieties about polio in complex and fascinating ways. This response runs the gamut from sensationalism and melodrama to lighthearted denial to the marked absence of polio texts in some quarters—specifically the total lack of an enduring literary canon before the mid-1970s and infrequent, idiosyncratic treatment of the topic in postwar women's magazines, where accurate, exhaustive coverage would have been most urgently sought after by mothers desperate to protect their children. Yet as interesting as are the textual gaps and effects created by widespread polio panic, they are problematic to the degree that their reflection of mainstream assumptions and prerogatives threatened then (and threatens now) the well-being of those Americans actually affected by polio in the postwar era and today. Many of the works to be discussed in this book tend to either overstate or understate polio's physical and psychological effects, mirroring the two modes of mistreatment of persons with serious illness or physical impairment perpetrated by the able-bodied mainstream: gaping with horror (often through sanctioned venues of voyeurism such as film and television) or completely ignoring the sick and impaired. That even polio-affected authors may be seen to perpetuate ableist assumptions to some extent is one more indicator of the pervasiveness of these assumptions as they control not only the literary marketplace but even the individual writing process, employed to produce the recognizable illness narrative.

As polio manifests as both an acute, life-threatening illness and, often, a life-long bodily transformation resulting in impairment of various kinds and degrees, the insights of both literature-and-medicine studies and disability studies guide this book's inquiry. The field of literature and medicine, well represented by Arthur Frank, quoted above, is noted for its focus on the patient's own narrative, often devalued in the medical setting yet often vital to the patient's self-reformation following a frightening diagnosis or a traumatizing illness experience. By contrast, disability studies sometimes takes a critical stance, placing little faith in the power of narrative to transform difficult physical situations, amassing evidence that shows a primarily adversarial relationship between the impaired person and the able-bodied mainstream who control the extramedical environment. In Rosemarie Garland Thomson's representative assessment, "Like the freak show . . . textual descriptions are overdetermined: they invest the traits, qualities, and behaviors of their characters with much rhetorical influence simply by omitting—and therefore erasing—other factors or traits that might mitigate or complicate the delineations. . . . Consequently, literary texts necessarily make disabled characters into freaks, stripped of normalizing contexts and engulfed by a single stigmatic trait."[14] Literature and medicine tends to personalize the narrative moment, reading the patient's own words as a liberating break from the vast impersonality of the medical system and describing one-on-one speaker/listener or writer/reader scenarios in which both producer and consumer of patient narrative are transformed. Some disability theorists by contrast look askance at the personalized scenario, at most efforts to privatize the problems of physical impairment with respect to the impaired person him or herself, or even, as for Thomson above, at the very structure of literary narrative. For these writers, solving the problems of disability is an expensive, complicated, but vital public responsibility; their focus is less on the doctor's office or the waiting room than on a broad social spectrum that includes inaccessible public spaces, discrimination in the workplace, and influential novels and films.

As persuasive as such sentiments may be, they are not universally shared within the disability studies ranks. Many, especially feminist disability theorists, distinguish a "social-modellist" approach, which may downplay both the individual narrative and the individual embodied therein, from their own attempt to integrate the individual and the collective (or the experiences of physical impairment and socially constructed "disability") in their work. While I appreciate this largely successful attempt to restore the role of narrative to disability studies, I am as indebted to narrative critique (provided by social model theorists) as I am to narrative embrace (provided by feminist disability theorists and literature-medicine theorists) in the course of my exploration of polio fiction and nonfictional accounts. Throughout this study I will interrogate the polio text in question for its ideologies of quarantine, ableism, and social division as well as its attempts to instruct, restore, and reintegrate both those untouched by the polio experience and those profoundly affected by it.

As polio's peak years in America occurred in the immediate postwar period, an era of re-entrenching gender polarities following the liberties allowed women during the war, issues of sex and gender further dimensionalize the discussion (or conflict) between the sick, the impaired, and the able-bodied outlined by the literature-medicine and disability theorists above. Postwar wives and mothers returned from the workforce to the home just when polio presented them with a (non-paying) job more difficult than any they had ever encountered at the factory or office: to protect their families from invisible armies of invading germs and pull their "brave little soldiers" safely through any polio infection. Women were both commissioned with the role of protecting families from polio or minimizing the fallout from such an attack *and* burdened with the responsibility when illness—ultimately through no fault of their own—befell the family. Of course, fathers of this period were equally at a loss to protect their children from the disease's dreaded visitations, and the crisis polio represented for both male and female parents will be analyzed here. Likewise, men and women's diverging styles of being polio *patients* —or, more specifically, the "masculine" and "feminine" approaches to illness and recovery exhibited by polio memoirists of both sexes—shed further light on the complications involved in representing polio most therapeutically for readers and writers themselves. Finally, of course, both men and women turned to medical science for answers that, for many, came too late, and sought ways to self-doctor their children and themselves, often through what they chose to read or write, in the days before the vaccine. Throughout, I will explore the masculine, feminine, ideological, and therapeutic properties of the phenomenon of denial, its several permutations within polio texts, and its relationship to other psychological responses to polio such as depression and acceptance.

The chapters are arranged by genre, four distinct modes of textual response to polio that have addressed different audiences and added to (or complicated) understanding of the subject in uniquely meaningful ways. I begin with one of the earliest forms of response, journalistic "coverage" in major women's magazines, although the quotes around the key term indicate that I am as interested in these publications' moments of genuine reporting on polio as I am in their attempts to cover over its tragedies, even its very existence. I move in the next chapter to another genre that boomed in the postwar era, although it is still in play today: the polio memoir, written by the polio survivor him or herself or a close friend or family member. My next chapter, on polio-related novels, analyzes a literary phenomenon distinct to the contemporary period; few polio novels were published in the United States before 1973. My fourth chapter moves back into the polio past—even the pre-war, Depression era—but investigates a genre that transitioned effectively from its mid-twentieth-century format (the rehabilitation center newsletter) to one well-suited to the contemporary moment (the lifestyle magazine for the physically impaired) and, since this is a genre that has renewed itself for each new generation of physically impaired Americans, has a certain timeless quality. The conclusion explores briefly a fifth mode of textual response—the postwar-era polio-related Hollywood film—briefly because, as with the postwar-era polio-related novel, this is a surprisingly small canon and because film, as the most widely "read" and thus often most influential cultural text, seemed the most fitting mode through which to explore the "big picture" of what polio has meant to American culture since its boom years in the postwar period.

The chapters arranged as they are will enable exploration of a conceptual chronology, alongside the historical one. For these respective polio genres are measurable in terms of the reader's own situation with respect to each, the position she is invited to occupy—before, within, or safely beyond polio's reaches—as she situates herself before the polio text in question. Postwar women's magazines reliably positioned their maternal readers safely (because permanently) *before* the polio specter, preaching a gospel of foresight and preparedness that was to translate for each reader into a polio-protected home. The polio memoir takes its reader, euphemistically or graphically, inside the polio experience, yet the majority also guide the reader safely back; the memoir-reading experience is often a journey *through* polio illness and rehabilitation and into sound health once more. Polio novels, largely by virtue of their recent publication dates, take readers into the polio past, an excursion profoundly affected by the reader's implicit understanding that, so many decades *after* the revolution effected by the Salk vaccine, polio is a world away. Like the polio memoir, both the polio newsletter and lifestyle magazine take the reader into the heart of the polio experience, but because this reader is much less often able-bodied and anxious than polio-affected, fully at home within the impairment experience, this mode of response is much less interested to move him or her to a false state of post-polio normality than to dwell *within* the polio/impairment experience, accompanying the reader through his or her daily living, just as does the impairment itself. The newsletter is in many ways a bracing corrective to the wealth of polio reporting and fiction-writing discussed in the preceding chapters, all of which presumes a mainstream, non-polio-affected readership.

To elaborate briefly, chapter 1, "'A Battle of Silence': Women's Magazines in the Postwar Polio Era," explores the range of approaches to polio taken by popular women's periodicals in the late 1940s and early 1950s. In it I analyze the surprisingly rare direct references to polio in the news coverage, features, and fiction in these magazines, as well as many moments of indirect reference employed, however inadvertently, in these same pages. Overt statements on polio often attempt to "frame" their most frightening elements with optimism, even humor, or consign the disturbing truth to the frame itself, that is, the textual margin. Conversely, indirect references suggest a polio subtext all the while they tell some other story: about a virus that "looks like POLIO," a girl on crutches with a curable condition, negligent parents in a short story whose children survive a threatening experience anyway. I argue that these various skirtings are as remarkable as overtly themed polio coverage in these magazines (if not more so), that they provided the reader a therapeutic exercise, from trauma to recovery, in a dry run for an actual occurrence that all fervently hoped would never actually occur.

In these magazines, I also locate a proto-feminist impulse that attested to women's capabilities as receivers and processors of frightening truths and straightforward medical information, even as these capabilities are questioned and undermined elsewhere in these same issues. Throughout, I evaluate the "battle of silence" (this chapter title comes from a polio-related article for a 1951 issue of *Redbook*) undertaken by these magazines, on behalf of women, with respect to polio: when was silence broken by direct discourse, and when and how did these publications' various silences prevent the sharing of necessary information?

Chapter 2, "'No Time for Tears'?: Gender, Fiction, and Denial in Polio Memoirs," considers the spate of polio nonfiction published in the immediate postwar period and followed up in recent decades with writings by long-time polio survivors. Assisted by the research and insight of multiple writers in disability studies and literature/medicine studies, I organize my response to these works along three lines of inquiry: gendered dimensions, the relationship between fiction and history, and the roles played by denial, depression, and acceptance. Reading gender in these works, I complicate an initial contrast between male and female polio memoirists with an analysis of "masculine" ("strong," "brave," "tough") approaches to the subject and "feminine" ("acquiescent," "enduring," "failed") ones, regardless of the sex of the auto/biographer or biographical subject. Noting that many polio narratives adopt a stance of strength through reliance on techniques of dismissal and denial, I determine that what we might characterize as the stereotypical manly response is often what is emotionally weakest, even as it remains of rich cultural value.

In this chapter, I discuss memoir's imbrications of fiction and history in texts whose testimonial status ("you, too, can catch polio and live to tell") went hand in hand with its role as recollection/report. Here I contend that those rendering obvious embellishments, glosses, and outright fabrications as "proof positive" are often those situated in denial, while those playing freely with fictional elements in otherwise fact-based accounts are those that move toward denial's opposite pole, acceptance. Finally, I consider texts that make detailed direct reference to the themes of denial, depression, and acceptance, noting that in these texts denial and acceptance are states of "happiness" notoriously difficult to distinguish, that each of these emotional states may be necessary, and necessarily revisited, in the course of polio rehabilitation and recovery. This chapter title is borrowed from Charles H. Andrews's early memoir of his son's "victory" over polio, a remarkable text that raises issues of gender roles, the testimonial value of polio nonfiction, and the detrimental aspects of denial.

Chapter 3, "'Crippled by History': Polio and the Past in Contemporary Novels," reads an array of long fiction from 1973 to the present, considering the strikingly late date of canon formation (1973 being almost two decades from the Salk vaccine), then exploring a significant resultant phenomenon: in America, the polio novel has almost always treated its subject as fully, irrevocably *past*, and polio's unique relationship to a "lost" (even golden) age of American innocence (1945–60), its unique ability to evoke this age (and pastness itself) for a variety of novelistic purposes, is the subject of this chapter. I relate the term "past" to the largely overlapping concept of "history," observing that the historical defines not only what has come and gone but also what authentically is or once was (as opposed to the fiction of historical inaccuracy, the fiction of novels themselves) and what is controlled by the vicissitudes of time and temporal measurement (as opposed to the elemental, the natural, the prelapsarian). All of these aspects of history are illuminated in their touching upon the specific example of polio in fiction treating the American past.

Analyzing a range of novels, from those considering personal or family histories affected by polio to those engaging with history writ large as this shapes and is shaped by polio and its survivors, I determine that polio is an incisive, revelatory index of the American past, even when the novels exploring this relationship fail as literature per se. To that end, I consider—and critique—two best selling fictions that take the misguided step of catapulting polio into a fantastic narrative future. This chapter's title comes courtesy of a key moment in James Carroll's *Secret Father* (2003) a novel effectively interimplicating major issues from twentieth-century American (and world) history: polio, World War II, the construction of the Berlin Wall, and the intrigue and eventual conclusion of the cold war.

Chapter 4, "'Heads, You Win!': Newsletters and Magazines of the Polio Nation," explores a genre of popular writing emerging from, perhaps originating from, the inpatient, rehabilitation, and outpatient experience of polio survivors: the chatty (even gossipy) newsletter, produced by and for the rehabilitation center residents themselves, that, in its very lightheartedness and triviality, enabled a form of therapeutic escape or release that nevertheless solidified each reader's bond with and identity within a specifically polio-oriented community. These newsletters adopted a range of verbal tones, visual styles, and thematic preoccupations, yet each is remarkably intimate, clubby, and vibrant. The close-knit, grassroots style on display in these early, brief, mimeographed circulars is even more remarkable when maintained—as it often was—as these in-house publications transformed into nationally (and internationally) distributed special interest magazines. These more professionalized serials kept close ties to local constituencies by exhorting them to read and contribute to each new issue by sending in their questions, comments, suggestions, or responses. Thus a dialogue was created among like-minded, like-situated crutch-, wheelchair-, or respirator-using "polios," who eventually united for political action when their vitally needed funding from the National Foundation declined and neither federal support nor societal awareness/acceptance were immediately forthcoming. While various of these publications professionalized to such a degree that they lost their grassroots quality (and, possibly, strength), each targeted a different sector of the polio community (including the "post-polio," able-bodied mainstream, who needed the most consciousness raising of all) and/or grew into a general disability-oriented publication (or online publication) reaching, connecting, and empowering ever wider audiences. This chapter's title topped a 1959 editorial from Gini Laurie, who cofounded a remarkable example in the genre of polio newsletter/magazines, the *Toomey j. Gazette*. The "heads" in question are Laurie's respirator-using readership; her remarkably strident reference characterizes the tough-minded irreverence of her "respo" audience and precedes her heartening reassurance that anyone who has survived polio with one's head intact—even if that is all one has left—has won an important victory and will continue, with the right outlook and the necessary support, to "win" such rewards.

My conclusion, "'The Voice is Still There': Some Final Notes on Postwar Polio Culture," focuses on three polio-related films from the postwar period, reading their patterns and unique contributions, considering their meanings for this larger project. The title comes from a pivotal moment in *Interrupted Melody* (1955), the story of opera star turned polio survivor Marjorie Lawrence, who after many months of debilitating depression relocates her voice—a preoccupation throughout this investigation of many remarkable silences surrounding polio. Here I note that film's many layers of representation call our attention to texts' own multi-dimensionality—a magazine story surrounded by illustrations, a polio memoir introduced by the first lady of the theater (and elsewhere, the first lady),[15] a heteroglossic contemporary novel of polio, and a polio newsletter produced by its own consumers—and sum up this project as a forging of relationship between polio voices and silences.

This book's title, *Bracing Accounts*, indulges in a bad pun that follows as best it can in the tradition of irreverent humor initiated by editor Laurie and the polio authors who have used a gallows sensibility to bring light and hope to the most difficult situations. Its reference to "accounts" signals once more this book's text-specific focus; its foregrounding of what is most "bracing" (embodied, assistive, literal, detailed, affecting, forthright, subversive, unforgettable) in each polio text examined for this study is meant to call simultaneously to mind the ways in which even those most weakly resolved to face this difficult subject head-on perform their bracing effects: supporting, sustaining, propping up the flagging spirits and failing bodies of their authors (and readerships) whose tendency in their writing toward fantasy and escape is largely understandable. Likely, the more bracing the account, the more fully the reader herself is "embraced" by the polio experience, either transported into a frightening moment from the American past or situated into the braces (or iron lung) of a writer for whom polio is still very much a present, ongoing circumstance. Such bracing accounts therefore not only provide an invaluable literary experience but raise consciousness among the complacent able-bodied and function as vital touchstones for polio (and other disability) communities.

1
"A Battle of Silence": Women's Magazines in the Postwar Polio Era

In the July 1950 issue of *Redbook*, an article entitled "The Town that Fought For Its Kids" (Fontaine) chronicles the polio epidemic that struck Muncie, Indiana, in the summer of 1949. It narrates the story of nurses and doctors at Ball Hospital who treated that summer's 120 polio cases, and of laborers who fashioned several iron lungs on extremely short order, all demonstrating the sort of selfless heroism typical for inspiring tales found in women's magazines of this period. But spoiling this upbeat mood, elsewhere in the story, fearful, desperate parents and spouses stand trapped behind glass viewing walls, smoke on the lawn outside, and pace the gallery while loved ones "fought for their lives" in isolation; in the opening moments a woman dies five days after becoming ill,[1] and mid-story a charming eight-year-old boy who struggles to survive in an iron lung also succumbs.[2]

While poliomyelitis, a paralyzing viral syndrome that struck children and young adults in record numbers throughout the immediate postwar period, might have been a topic of chief interest in a magazine such as *Redbook*, aimed almost entirely at young mothers, in fact its direct address, as in the article described here, was a rare occurrence in multiple top women's publications from the late 1940s to the mid-1950s, when the Salk and Sabin vaccines were perfected. Strikingly, these magazines' chief purpose seems to have been to guide women in the process of ignoring, denying, or forgetting the anxieties that attended motherhood during this period, especially during the dreaded summer months when polio incidents almost always dramatically increased. While such fears were everywhere in waking existence — and referred to frequently in news magazines such as *Time*, *Newsweek*, and *Life* magazines—women's popular periodicals favored stories of progress and triumph in polio when they mentioned the issue at all.[3]

In fundamental ways, women's magazines positioned readers *before* the specter of polio, in keeping both with their stressing of common sense and total preparedness as universal approaches to wife- and motherhood, and also, paradoxically, with their role as entertainment, even escapist literature for women. The inveterate lightheartedness that as a matter of course characterized each issue simulated the relief and elation of successfully avoided tragedy: not my child, not this summer, not in my backyard. Media historian Nancy A. Walker notes a boom in advice columns in women's magazines in the postwar period[4] and argues that this represented "both a continuing professionalization of the role of the homemaker and a national faith in scientific advancement to improve domestic life and help wage the Cold War."[5] As its main mission was the arming of women with the information necessary to successfully maintain a marriage, home, and children, its implicit universal theme of "What to do if . . ." became in the polio context a mantra that implicitly equated preparedness with prevention. Positioning polio always in the reader's future, the women's magazines of this era presented endlessly staved-off disaster: polio may be here tomorrow but within the bounds of these ultimately escapist publications, tomorrow almost never came. Those maternal readers who unfortunately became polio mothers during this period, crossing from "pre-" to "intra-polio" status, were simply no longer the magazines' primary target of address. Instead, they spoke perforce almost solely to the fearful but hopeful pre-polio mother, situating her safely because perpetually before the tragedy of polio.

In this chapter, four leading women's magazines of the period—*Good Housekeeping*, *Ladies Home Journal*, *McCall's*, and *Redbook*—are considered; while the entrenched traditionalism of the first three may explain several of the textual effects to be considered in this discussion, even the relatively progressive, "young adult" orientation of *Redbook* did not enable a noticeably more forthright handling of the subject of polio. Certainly, mid-century gender politics account at least in part for such omissions: the editorial boards of these women's publications were at least half male, with men occupying all of the top editor and publisher positions, and the assumption that women had no interest in or stomach for realistic news coverage may not surprise us.[6] Additionally, the example of the most famous polio-affected person in America, FDR, who enjoyed a productive public life by largely ignoring his impairment may have set the example of genteel circumspection that publishers of "ladies'" magazines sought to emulate.[7] Finally, silence on this subject may also have stemmed from the tradition of grinning and bearing perpetuated by Americans of both sexes and all ages who had survived the Depression and Second World War. Yet despite the attempt to minimize the worst that polio represented to American women, these publications signified the crisis anyway: in their rare direct references to the issue, in their telling omissions and circumventions, and in their raising the issue of women's ability to maintain family health and safety.

In each case, the editorial approach to its audience is ambivalent: bad news about polio (the direct address) is insistently minimized, couched in optimistic, even frivolous terms; writing on serious medical subjects often "looks like" polio but turns out to be something harmless, while in writing on nonmedical but no less suggestive subject matter (children, summer, the waterfront), the obvious threat posed by polio is consistently ignored; and the magazines' frequent endorsement of women's ability to care for and protect is undermined by opinions held elsewhere in these same publications. With respect to polio news and information, we sense the danger of this ambivalent approach: if women had insufficient or incorrect information, they may have enacted the wrong protective measures or failed to do anything at all. If trusted advisors (i.e., the magazines themselves) questioned women's native intelligence and their ability to learn new skills, children were endangered (if not from polio than from uncertain mothers) yet again. I am suggesting, therefore, that the mixed signals sent by women's publications, while certainly not guilty of exposing its audience or their families to polio, in important ways "paralyzed" and "disabled" its maternal readership at the moment when it was most desperate to act decisively and effectively against a dangerous biological adversary.

It has been well documented that women during the polio era understood the magnitude of the problem and worked productively against it. Jane S. Smith details the multi-level structure of the National Foundation for Infantile Paralysis, whose battalions of volunteers in every county and city were "manned" in large part by women. Mothers were especially famous for their house-to-house search for donors to the annual March of Dimes campaign and came from multiple ethnic and social backgrounds to gather and disseminate information, collect funds for the Foundation, staff offices, and provide comfort to grieving families.[8] In addition were the countless female nurses and physical therapists treating polio patients daily, and at the top of their respective professions: the

Australian nurse Elizabeth Kenny, who developed a method of physical rehabilitation that saved many a spastic limb from permanent paralysis; Oveta Culp Hobby, FDR's secretary of Health and Human Services; pioneer vaccine researcher Isabel Morgan;[9] and Virginia Blood, Dorothy Ducas, Elaine Whitelaw, and Bea Wright, key players in the highest ranks of the National Foundation. In the polio period women mobilized as productively as they did during WWII when factories lost their male workforce and women rushed to fill the need. In separate texts, Elaine Tyler May and Steven Mintz/Susan Kellogg document the phenomenon of displaced women who found themselves frustrated and bored at war's end when husbands returned and reoccupied their former professions,[10] while the magazines themselves tell the story of a revolution in housekeeping technology during this period that freed up women's time in unprecedented ways. For all its horrors, the polio crisis gave women a role to play, and women lent tremendously to the alleviation of its difficulties in the years before the vaccine.

Framing the Problem

Certainly direct references to polio occur on occasion in women's magazines of this time. "The Girl Who Never Gave Up" tells of an attractive young woman, skillful enough with a paintbrush (held precariously in her polio-affected hand) to look forward to a successful art career.[11] Elsewhere, a review of recent polio research is accompanied by a close-up of a beautiful little girl, facing us from the bed of her iron lung, looking scared, not "brave."[12] A triumphant narrative of the Salk vaccine trials in the *Journal* brings so much thunder-stealing optimism to this era's penultimate chapter that the utter lack of polio coverage by this same magazine in 1955 (the year the vaccine succeeded) is almost not surprising.[13] Yet each of these reports frames its bad news (sometimes literally) with insistent optimism, or attempts to relegate what is most disturbing about its story *to* the framing apparatus, to the margins where it can be bracketed from central focus. Meanwhile, these framing techniques fail to obscure persisting fears, contradictions, and unanswered questions.

The photo of the frightened little girl, for instance, clashes with the optimism of the title of Margaret Clark's article, "Polio is Being Defeated." The text itself also runs counter to this promise: in fact, the author only surveys the fits and starts that have defined the research process; while the "dynamic young bacteriologist" Jonas Salk is a featured player, he has no breakthroughs to report, as the vaccine is still two years away.[14] Disturbing images undermine the upbeat intent of "The House that Kindness Built" as well.[15] A town-spirit piece reminiscent of "The Town that Fought For Its Kids," its equally innocuous, all-purpose title celebrates the can-doism of local craftsman and the object of their charity, respirator-using Mary Kitsmiller. Through the mirror attached to her iron lung, we see Mary's sunny smile; despite "moods" of "depression" and "gloom," in the final paragraph she is "supremely happy" and feels like shouting "God bless everyone!"[16] The accompanying photos, meanwhile, cannot help but disturb: while we learn that Mary can spend eight hours a day with a portable respirator, she is only seen prostrate and fully encased within a tank respirator—making a phone call with her son's help; watching television (backward, through her mirror); having dinner, backed up to the table, with her son and parents (her husband has run off); receiving an awkward hug from her boy who can only clutch at her head. As Mary's own situation is a mixture of "gloom" and "happiness," so the images themselves attempt to put the best face on difficult circumstances with only mixed results.

Good Housekeeping considers "Your Child's Camp and POLIO" and to open provides a quote from an exuberant health official with the National Foundation: "Is it safe to send your child to camp? Yes!"[17] Summer camp was always a concern, since it involved the transfer of children from one setting to another, where viral strains unfamiliar to a child's immune system might lurk. Yet despite the initial reassurance, it is later revealed that the best a camp can do is care adequately for a child once s/he takes sick; to elaborate, a camp that badly handled a polio outbreak is contrasted with one that successfully controlled hysteria. Later, the author acknowledges that "no one knows how infantile paralysis is communicated,"[18] no one understands routes of transmission, and "none of the phenomena of the [summer] season—heat, humidity, summer foods, etc.—has been proved to contribute to polio's spread."[19] Only slightly more than half the New England camps surveyed responded to a questionnaire about their polio histories, and those that did provide statistics that are "inconclusive."[20] Despite the optimistic "yes!" that opened this discussion, persisting questions make such reassurances far from reassuring.

Three months later, *Good Housekeeping*'s Maxine Davis labors to assure her readership with comforting data: "statistics show that not many people in a total population get polio in any one year," and "If a person is infected, *the chances are that he will not be seriously crippled or die.*"[21]

Parents and school officials are instructed to send children to school *during* polio outbreaks, and again this may have seemed like irresponsible advice. The author recommends "isolation in bed of all patients with fever, pending diagnosis"[22] but directly across the page lists "Isolation" and "Quarantine" among "Unnecessary and Useless Precautions";[23] quarantining infected families is described as "hysterical" community behavior in one paragraph and as "common sense" in the next.[24] Shall we read these happy headlines as irresponsible journalism in light of the grim details and myriad contradictions, acknowledged and unacknowledged, in the fine print? Or were such comforting messages necessary couchings of bad news that parents had every right be eased through as therapeutically as possible? Indeed, the mysteries surrounding polio's many paths of infection—in water, milk, or flies? through the respiratory or digestive tract? in my city this summer or next?—that were only beginning to be understood must have made the task of giving information, advice, or assurance as fraught with difficulties as receiving it.

Yet elsewhere, this framing technique is so inappropriately employed that it verges on the truly tasteless. Near the end of the Davis piece, medical authority concedes that "the disease is on the rise" and describes "the crippling aftereffects of the disease [that] follow the death of or damage to the nerve cells."[25] Cultural theorists like John Berger have pointed to the jarring juxtaposition of frivolous advertising surrounding stories of tragedy and disaster;[26] on the pages in question here, flexible shank oxfords named "Lazy-Bones" ensure "healthy, normal feet" to the right of the article, and far left a girl measures her little sister's upright posture against a measuring stick on the wall. Two even more curious examples are human interest "items" about polio, bordered by charming curlicues and effectively bracketed by the frivolous material surrounding them: a "Polio Pledge" occupies the upper right quadrant of a page continuing the short story "It's Always Some Man!,"[27] and the tiny insert "If Polio Strikes My Home" floats incongruously in a sea of soup recipes from "Our Young Marrieds."[28] Do these heterogeneous layouts indicate a readership so "at home" with polio that references found anywhere were expected, thus appropriate? Or do they bespeak an editorial discomfort so acute that efforts to hide, disguise, and sugarcoat the medicine spoon of polio discourse resulted inevitably in such erratic and bizarre presentations?

Earlier I indicated that even Fontaine's "Town that Fought" piece silences some aspects of its polio story with respect to its optimistic, all-purpose title. It is Fontaine who coined the phrase that names the chapter in progress here, as he described the town's realization that the epidemic was upon them: "[I]t was a battle against panic as much as polio. And it was a battle of silence, save for the occasional screaming of a siren through the streets, of waiting, of self-control, and of courage repeatedly renewed."[29] Later he notes the "quiet compulsion of fear" characterizing the talk of the waiting parents and the "stoicism" of the country wife that only occasionally gives way to "sobbing."[30] An accompanying montage illustration is also "silent" in its depiction of children or patients of any kind; instead nurses and doctors consult, mother's proffer donation cans, workmen make adjustments to an unoccupied iron lung. Elsewhere, the silences kept even by public figures are yet more remarkable: the polio bout of the eldest son of Don McNeill (host of the phenomenally popular radio program *The Breakfast Club*) is largely confined to the caption of single photo—of the son in perfect health—in a story about the show and its warm-hearted cast and audience,[31] while Helen Hayes narrates the story of her daughter's death from polio without a single mention of the word.[32] Would less stoicism and more sobbing in stories like these have spread lifesaving awareness, or at least comforted those most seriously affected, whose mandate to bear up under such circumstances must have made the suffering only worse? The townsfolk of Muncie, the author of their story, and the editors who published it, along with producers of multiple similar texts, seemed to have felt otherwise.

Skirting the Issue

Thus, writings that directly referenced polio were careful to frame the problem with the perennial silver lining or to build a solid, however incongruous, wall of silence around it. Meanwhile, dozens more writings, seemingly unrelated to the subject of polio, indeed skirt this issue in one of two ways:[8] 1) with loaded language that fizzles into less serious, even frivolous, themes; and 2) with fixations on subject matter distinctly proximal to the polio crisis itself—medicine, children (and the combined issue of sick or imperiled children), and summertime (a theme that also almost always suggested children).

Certainly sensationalism is a staple of much of the fiction and feature writing in all the publications surveyed here. Story titles and illustrations hint at torrid affairs and violent crimes that turn out to be only imagined or dreamt; doctors' advice comes urgently accented in bold print but refers to treatable problems like gallbladder infection or hemorrhoids. An article entitled "Mother, Beware"[33] turns out to be a bit of nonsense about a little girl crying because her ponytail is too tight, while another called "What to do in a PANIC"[34] (*Good Housekeeping*/Porter) raises the issue of a sick child only to discuss the "panic" of paying hospital expenses. While certainly such expenses are of concern, and certainly the cost of polio care and rehabilitation would have bankrupted thousands of families had it not been for the financial support of the March of Dimes, the "scare" over expenses pales in comparison to the terror induced by the child's illness itself. The "false alarm" subtext of such alarmist features may have had therapeutic value for mothers who lived in fear of realized or unrealized medical catastrophe. Indeed, picturing oneself surviving a devastating experience is an exercise suggested by grief and trauma counselors even today; these panicky headlines that turn out to be nothing may have led women through just such a picturing exercise whether reader or writer recognized this or not.

Rarely was fatal illness addressed in these publications (though *Redbook* bucked the trend with features on cancer and TB), with a remarkable exception from a doctor who defended his right to lie to patients with hopeless conditions.[35] Luckily, "The Disease that Imitates POLIO" turns out to be Coxsackie virus, a much more benign virus of childhood,[36] while three doctors in St. Petersburg host a series of town meetings whose most burning issues are the common cold, hypertension, and allergies.[37] Without evidently a mention of polio during this multiweek series, the event is deemed by its author an enjoyable success, complete with doctors cracking jokes about "egg-zema" during the proceedings. In one of his regular columns for *Redbook*, Leo Smollar, M.D., promises readers "It Won't Kill You!," leaving the business of defining "it"—hypochondria—for the ninth paragraph of the article.[38] Elsewhere, singer Jane Froman is pictured clowning around with Milton Berle with a brace on her right leg.[39] She is revealed to be recovering from a harrowing plane crash from which she was heartwarmingly rescued by the pilot she later married.

Even columns focused on children's health primarily field questions about Junior's moping, bedwetting, or other emotional troubles, and while such issues deserve coverage, the child's ultimately sound health is always affirmed.[40] (Often the problem is attributed not to a child's physical or emotional debility but to mother's nagging, and it is easy to read the copious "advice" in these several features simply as criticism.[41]) Feature articles about sick children emphasize perseverance, pluck, and recovery; while wheelchairs, braces, crutches, and convalescent beds are regular components of such narratives and their accompanying photos, with one exception noted above (i.e., "The Girl Who Never Gave Up"), the problem is *not* polio. In the *Journal*, six- or seven-year-old Karen is pictured in a small inset with the brace/crutch apparatus universally identified with post-polio ambulation, yet the anxiety provoked by such an image is immediately relieved by the full-page photo at left of slightly older Karen bounding independently up a flight of stairs.[42] Shortly into the narrative the trouble is connected to Karen's exceeding prematurity—she was two pounds at birth—not polio. What is eventually diagnosed as Karen's cerebral palsy can be read as a false alarm only by the reader, spared this time from having to consider these debilities rooted in a dreaded contagious virus like polio and spared being "infected" by the haunting question, "what if my child is next?"

In a robust counterstatement to the polio-at-camp piece referred to above, Floyd Miller exclaims that "Camp is *Good* For 'Em!,"[43] and the only camper to take sick in the course of the article suffers from hypochondria's first cousin, "psychosomaticism." In a photo feature, "A Boy's Summer," nine-year-old Tim Gaillard leads a charmed life, with only a "summer cold" brought on by an "all-afternoon swim"[44] to slow him down; when a children's health column describes "Summer Problems,"[45] polio danger themes like trips to the country, overheating, and swimming present only their benign aspects: poison ivy, sunburn, fear of the water. Polio's status as living-room elephant in these examples bespeaks the paralyzing fear polio evoked in this period; the audience in St. Petersburg could not bring itself to articulate its most pressing question, and even science writers and physician-columnists, commissioned to write about the dangers of childhood, flinched at the mandate to address what was clearly foremost in every mother's mind. Yet ultimately, I argue, each of the examples discussed here "imitates polio" in significant ways: as Coxsackie bears an uncanny clinical and virological resemblance to dreaded poliomyelitis, so the article discussing it quickens readerly anxiety as it seeks to allay this—by detailed description of a viral complex that, if anything else, is at least not polio. As these several writings move as close as possible to directly referencing the issue of fatal illness, specifically polio, without ever actually naming it, polio's profound ability to infect the cultural imagination, even at great distances, ensures their supplemental status as "about polio" nevertheless.

At Water's Edge

The '50s-era seen-but-not-heard generation of children were both seen and heard in the pages of these magazines as they rarely are in contemporary issues of these same publications. The "Mother, Beware" article referred to above was one of several features *on* children's hairstyles, while children's and teen's clothing and shoes received multipage layouts at least once or twice a year. *McCall's* popular "Betsy McCall" was both a line of children's clothing regularly featured in the magazine's advertising section and a paper cutout complete with several fashions to snip and attach (for the kids, of course); mother-daughter dresses were a popular component of sewing-based fashion spreads. Infants, school-age children, and teens received regular attention in feature articles, while the entirety of *Redbook*—pitched toward "young adults"—likely expected a large contingent of teen readers. Teens asked for and doled out advice, discussed their parents in photo-filled essays, and wrote letters to the editor. "Children's pages" with puzzles, rhymes, and drawings were provided in many issues, and of course cute babies and small children were a staple in countless advertisements. These serials' covers also provided a context for youth images; *Good Housekeeping* depicted children exclusively on its covers throughout the years surveyed, while the "surprised baby" offered a whimsical touch—especially at holiday time—on the covers of *McCall's* and *Ladies Home Journal*. Of course the intense child-orientation of these magazines reflects the equally obsessive family-focus of its readership and, again, marks them as ideal venues for frequent, straightforward coverage of polio that is instead largely absent.

Most striking of all are the children's covers for the summer issues of these magazines, which almost inevitably picture the child beside a body of water. The swimming pool and public beach were feared hotbeds of polio infection during the summers of epidemic years, when mothers anguished daily over whether to keep their children home or let them enjoy their freedom. Can images of pools and beachfronts, however idyllically rendered, have failed to strike a frightening chord in the subconscious or conscious understanding of these maternal readers? The editorial decision to position so many children blithely poised at the edge of the abyss seems remarkably insensitive. August was usually a high-water mark (no pun intended) in polio infections each year, yet the August 1950 issue features an infant propped on her chubby forearms at the crashing water's edge. We know she is at the very shoreline because her reflection in the sand beneath her indicates a sheen of water from the recently receded tide. The sense of postponed but inevitable danger, realized with the next forward surge of the waves, reflects the larger issue of children imperiled by summers at the beach during this period. Ironically, a banner across the top of this cover advertises the "First Complete Handbook on Infantile Paralysis," included as a special supplement.[46]

The year 1952 holds the record for polio cases in America, yet this did not prevent *Good Housekeeping* from offering a chilling July cover. Here a small blond girl, hands folded prayer-style, arcs from a diving board into a pool. The child's prayerful attitude suggests her fervent wish to be spared the scourge of polio this year, while rare was the mother who trusted prayer alone, without a full complement of hygienic habits, precautions, and cleaning products in support. If we presume this child's relative safety because she is alone in this setting, the solitude itself suggests disturbing questions: are the other children missing because their mothers know better? because they fear the pictured child's potential infectiousness? because they have already succumbed to illness, leaving this last little survivor to spend the summer by herself? From a sufficiently aware perspective—one that, I argue, all mothers would have had access to, whether they engaged it or not—this pleasant, cheering image is grimly undermined. That such covers appeared dependably for many summers indicates that their potential offensiveness did *not* ever hit home; even at the height of the polio period, summer's traditional "escapist" associations evidently encouraged mothers to escape their summertime anxieties through these images, and enabled publishers to escape the charge of unethical journalism.

Summer Stories

Summertime, socially unconventional adults, and children narrowly avoiding physical or emotional disaster are a recurring thematic combination in fiction offerings throughout these pages. As noted above, the theme of summer suggests the presence of children engaged in warm-weather leisure activities and likewise invites adult figures to indulge in escapist "vacations" from the ordinary rules of spousal and parental behavior. In these stories, the adult characters change locations permanently or temporarily, alone and in secret or with family in tow, threaten the emotional or physical well-being of those around them with their selfish acts, and function as neglectful parent figures whether they have biological offspring or not. In short, they act up, misbehave, run away from home, and carry on *like children*; conversely, the children often display remarkably mature behaviors, caring for the adults in the midst of (and in spite of) their childish midlife crises, bearing the burden of the adults' mistakes, and even taking the blame for these.[47] Complicating matters further, young adult characters who occupy the middle ground between child- and adulthood function frequently as overgrown children, disrupting family structures that rest on two distinct generations and enticing the parental figures to misbehave even more outlandishly. While the stories to be surveyed here range in genre from silly comedy to sappy romance to near-tragedy, all take part in this discussion and share the theme of summer's particularity—when all rules give way.

I read these suggestive themes for their pertinence to the "real" story that may be seen to lurk beneath—of failed parenting, familial betrayal, and threatened or lost lives all enacted within the polio context of the time. While certainly little to nothing could have been done to ensure a child's (or young adult's) health, parents—especially mothers?—no doubt felt crushed by guilt and remorse at a child's positive diagnosis. Ruminations about what might have been done differently and recriminations between adult family members were surely the topics of anguished dialogues (or never-spoken monologues), and the urge to "make up" to the afflicted family member—for lost time, lost happiness, lost chances to love better—is addressed in these stories of parents who get second chances and children who emerge from danger physically and emotionally unscathed. In fact, these children function, in their spirited, generous ability to rebound from any troubling situation, as ideal polio patients: brave little soldiers who surmount fear and pain with smiles on their faces. The reversals and reunions of junior and senior family members, as these constitute the conflicts and resolutions in these stories, comment importantly on family roles during the polio era.

In the frothy confection, "Frothingham," the eponymous character is a nosey but brainy kid, sent to summer camp by parents who, according to the wise-cracking narrator, "could not face another whole summer" with their pesky, curious son.[48] I discussed above the anxieties plaguing parents regarding the issue of summer camps in the polio period, and in its early pages, the story plays fast and loose with the suggestive occurrence of a new, pretty nurse arriving at camp, who has everyone, young adult counselors and boy children, lined up for medicine at the infirmary: "Before she had a chance to take off her hat, a long line of counselors and campers, seeking immediate medical attention for headaches and fevers [the classic first symptoms of polio], had formed outside the infirmary door. 'Who am I to complain?' [the narrator asks]. 'But I think the rate of sickness at Camp Okodochee this summer will be alarming.'"[49] As the children play the disturbing role of "sick campers" and share precociously in the college boys' sexual interest in the new nurse, so children and adults trade parts in the story, creating the comedy that ensues: the grown-ups get caught up in foolish games of gossip and intrigue, while young Frothingham solves disputes and reunites the estranged Sam and Lily through his persistent questions and independent action.

In another just-as-silly tale, "The Fair-Weather Kind," parents Brad and Jody move their kids from urban to suburban LA and are then hounded by city friends who monopolize the pool and ruin the kids' sleep schedule; pathos is generated by the many selfish errors committed by the parents before realizing that "our kids are people, too."[50] Little Ricky and Linda bravely tolerate being ignored and shunted from the pleasant poolside back indoors, even offering at one point to play in the sandbox instead. In "Free as a Gull" Johnny restores his father's devastated ego by referring to his bout with unconsciousness, due to a disastrous boat trip that lands them both in the water during a violent storm, as "falling asleep."[51] He awakes with a smile and a string of insignificant questions about a lost fishing rod that reassure his parents of no trauma or resentment post-incident. In both stories, the juvenile maturity and generosity embarrass the adults; Jody "wished that [her children] had had a tantrum. Anything but that painfully adult acceptance of [Brad's] rejection,"[52] while Johnny's father Bill, reacting to his son's claim to have fallen asleep "hadn't known that words could cause such actual physical pain."[53] The discomfort is succeeded by gratitude, however, when the adults realize that in fact the children have healed the parents and saved the family from falling apart.

Just as chatty Frothingham was displaced to summer camp—by parents who set their own needs above his—so in "Fair-Weather" and "Free as a Gull" parents remove kids from city to country for everyone's benefit only to learn that their citified entanglements leave them ill-equipped to fend off hazards to their children in this new environment: Jody and Brad move to a far-flung LA suburb for the sake of the kids, then miss old friends who wind up exploiting their summer invitations, while Bill's city-slickerism prevents him from correctly reading weather conditions on the day of the fateful boat trip. While Bill's son nearly dies—by exposure to dangerous waters—before Bill learns the lesson of his limitations, Brad and Jody see their error and recoup their kids' loss by *pre-*

venting them from going near the water. They devise a plot to outwit their selfish friends, and the reader presumes this will involve the children finally having access to their own pool. In fact, the family revisits the city where in various friends' cramped apartments the kids break vases and order large breakfasts at early hours until the light dawns on each offending couple. While at first glance this is yet another case of parents acting primarily in their own interest, from the "polio" perspective, they act on their children's behalf—by resolving the larger privacy issue while protecting the little ones from the dangers that pools may have posed at the time.

Two stories that deal explicitly with polio are even more instructive on this issue of unconventional (or failed) parenting. Beginning with its plainly suggestive title, "Dangerous Summer" moves immediately to references to two characters with physical disabilities: Professor Charles Neill who is "lame," and Aunt Sophy who sprains her ankle and cannot accompany niece Eve to tea with the professor, clearing the way for their romance.[54] Eve follows a limb-threatening "rough footpath" up to the professor's home, and after the tea she watches in alarm as the professor's son Chip threatens his own life and limb "traversing a tree branch [or limb] like a cat."[55] As Charles's limp is in fact a result of polio in his childhood, so Aunt Sophy seems to have "caught" her sprained ankle from the professor's contagious condition; no sooner does she mention his game leg than she "comes down" with one herself, while both Eve and Chip come into harm's way but never show visible signs of "infection," resembling the countless polio cases in this period believed by doctors to have subsided after initial flu-like symptoms.

In the "polio" reading of this story, Chip's moment of acrobatics on the tree branch is its most resonant event. The act provokes in Eve a look of accusation toward permissive Father, who defends against the charge of possibly infecting his son with his own lame condition by arguing, "but I want him to be happy and free of fear."[56] His desire to see Chip active and fearless indicates his generous willingness to let his son outstrip him physically, yet also points to the distance separating the energetic boy and his middle-aged, physically limited father. For while the professor is dashing and distinguished, dances divinely, and turns out to be quite the romantic after all, his busy schedule at the university and reserved external manner mark him as distinctly unsuited for the raising of a small boy. He is in fact too busy to take Chip to the circus he is longing to see, whose high-wire act he had been imitating on the branch. If Chip is to gratify his free-spiritedness with a visit to the aerialist Madam

Raj, Eve will have to enmesh herself in family politics by escorting the boy herself: "she had come to the country to find peace and escape from the demands of other people. Yet now here she was, involved."[57] This initial "involvement," contiguous with the path of "infection" I have been tracing thus far, foreshadows her later dilemma regarding whether to return to her career as globe-trotting photojournalist or to trade in this physical mobility for a much more settled life with Charles and Chip.

Throughout, Eve's romance with Charles is figured explicitly in terms of a polio-like illness: upon meeting, "neither of them moved,"[58] paralyzed with love at first sight in accordance with the dictates of the story's romance genre. Unnerved by her infatuation, Eve is "stiff" at first, then "stumbles" toward her car at the end of the date, reacting to the professor's intense parting glance.[59] In the throes of attraction—and of grief for her dying career—"a sick fear overcame her";[60] she endures "brittle patter" and "leaden silence" as she dissembles with Charles,[61] responds "limply" to her boss on the phone from New York, and speaks "feverishly" to Chip at the circus, who asks "'You sick, Ms. Ankerstone?' . . . eyeing her exhausted face."[62] Contagion spreads once more in the circus scene, when moments later it is announced that Madam Raj is sick and cannot perform that day, causing Chip to cry out with despair "in a strangled voice."[63] Following the disappointment, Eve speaks to Chip with "infinite weariness," then returns home to Aunt Sophy where she experiences "a sort of malaise."[64]

The story's climactic moment, Eve's giving in to love, begins with a striking momentary shift from romance to horror: "She fumbled for her key and looked up, a set speech on her lips, to see Charles standing several feet away. There was a curious threat in the dark, still figure. . . . [H]e was coming toward her, each step echoing through the hot, scented night. He did not hurry. Almost, she thought, as if I could not run away and he knew that. Her eyes closed."[65] While the story deserves commendation for its subversive figuring of women's professional self-sacrifice in terms of violent, mortal threat, the demonizing of the afflicted Charles is unfortunate. His characterization at this moment recalls the findings of disability film theorists Martin Norden, Robert Bogdan, and others, who critique a long tradition of assigning bogey men physical deformities to increase their frightfulness to the able-bodied viewer. By the end of this scene, which ends in the inevitable clinch, Charles is restored to his role as dashing romantic hero, yet by story's end, he will have transferred his ineffable stillness to Eve, who is successfully enjoined to acknowledge her destiny and settle permanently in the rural South, her earlier statement, that "I'd die shut away in this valley where nothing happens,"⁶⁶ echoing eerily.

In several of these stories, children settle disagreements between adults, bringing parents or parent figures together; here, the "danger" Chip is in—if not of falling from a tree branch than of being parented solely by a middle-aged man unable to keep up with him—causes Eve to realize both motherly and wifely instincts. Her decision to be "on vacation" permanently at story's end—to transform the seasonal "dangers" of summer into a permanent condition for herself and her limping family—is countered by our recognition that in fact Eve saves her new son from "polio"—from his father's limited, post-polio condition that would likely have spelled a sadder, narrower life for him—as all good mothers should.⁶⁷ Interestingly, she saves him from this polio-affected fate by becoming hobbled herself, a gesture of atonement the story implicitly suggests is in order for Eve's ultimately transgressive attempt to choose career over marriage.

The illustration accompanying "Summer Bachelor" depicts a gray-templed man leaning over a steamy young blond, suggesting yet another enlargement of the adults-making-mischief theme I have explored throughout this discussion. Sure enough, Cowan Matthews summers alone at the country club while his wife Anne is away, and the "kid" he takes up with there is explicitly positioned as a generation-straddling third element who brings out in Cowan both the red-hot lover and questionable cradle-robber. Betty has a "little boarding-school voice" and turns out to be "Ed Durston's daughter,"⁶⁸ although she is primarily the homewrecking siren in this characterological triangle, while Cowan's father role rests in neutral in the absence of his biological child Donny. Immediately into the story, these logistics are strikingly complicated: in fact, Ann and Donny have left Cowan on his own because "there had been a frightening increase in the polio epidemic [near the country club] in the last few weeks, and . . . Anne was going to take [Donny] over to a lodge near [his summer] camp and stay a week or two until the epidemic had quieted down."⁶⁹ If Cowan's failure to join Anne in her effort to protect their son did not reflect negatively enough upon his character, his indulgence in lazy afternoons at the beach, flirtations with young women, and card games with the club's notorious wife-swapping set, while Anne and Donny sweat it out in the "even hotter" summer camp setting,⁷⁰ suggests his thorough unworthiness as a parent. In fact, it is this level of negligence that might be held to blame in the case of an infected child, and this midlife-crisis romance that turns out to also be a story about polio raises fascinating questions about the issue of parental culpability in an epidemic moment.

Significantly, Anne's letter to Cowan early in their separation expresses less "worry about contagion"[71] for Donny than for Cowan and his tendency to fall in with the wrong crowd in her absence. She explicitly advises avoiding the sexually unconventional Carstairses, yet in fact Cowan becomes "infected" with their fast-living ways when he pursues Betty more and more avidly during afternoons at the beach. Of course the lovers' beach setting is affected by the story's pervasive polio theme; recall that Betty is still a "kid," a young adult almost equally likely to be infected with polio in the mid-'50s (when the virus tended to strike older age groups), and thus endangered by her beach exposure, again by Cowan, who draws her to the water's edge day after day. The water is described as "amazingly cold," while the sun "rays bit[ing] into [Cowan's] chest,"[72] Betty's "tan skin,"[73] and the couple's mutual sexual attraction figure Cowan and Betty as "overheated"; significantly, exposure of overheated youngsters to "very cold water" is cited by at least one author of a monthly children's health column for *The Journal* as a major gateway to polio infection.[74] Almost inevitably the beach is "crowded," while a seemingly innocent moment contains chilling undertones: "At the water's edge the nurses already had established themselves, starched Nannies in linen sunshade hats, watching their toddler charges splash about in the shallows. The children and a timid lady in water to her waist were the only ones sharing the ocean with him."[75]

At last seeking an end to dissipation, Cowan summons Anne and Donny to join him, yet his attempt to resume the role of respectable spouse and father is not only questionable for its basic inertia—why, in fact, does he not leave the country club to join his family instead?—but also for its being rooted in a dangerous lie. "What about the epidemic?" Anne asks when he calls. "Wasn't there a case in the village just last week?" "Oh, *that*," is Cowan's unconscionable brush-off. "There's no epidemic here. Just talk. Besides, Donny would be a lot happier down here at the beach."[76] At this most remarkable of cultural intersections the story presents its readership with what at that time was a true moral dilemma: is the extramarital affair so depraved an act that it is acceptable to risk a child's health to avoid it? In fact, the story's final movements play daringly with the potential seriousness of Cowan's lie. A day after his call to Anne, Cowan hears about the "County Judge's kid" who died of polio two days after coming down with it. Anne and Donny both arrive "exhausted" with Anne complaining of the heat and refusing to go near the beach, and Donny "collapsing slackly" into a rocking chair.[77] That evening, Donny comes down with a headache and fatigue and his parents are terrified.

But in a move that returns us to the comforting distance of polio metaphors and analogues, Cowan leaves Anne to wait for Donny's doctor while he himself goes to the country club dance to break things off with Betty. At the party, he is "sickened by" the reveling wife-swappers, seeming to take on his son's illness in a gesture of healing atonement—recall this identical dynamic between Eve and Chip above—and overcomes his desire for Betty in a final leave-taking that confirms for the reader his moral soundness. This "clean break" is evidently all that is needed to redeem himself and his son; upon his return, Donny's symptoms have been diagnosed as a "slight summer cold,"[78] and Cowan's child-imperiling selfishness can be forgiven and forgotten. While this story in particular treats polio even as it considers larger issues regarding marriage, parenting roles, and the "innocence" of "kids," each of those considered here comments meaningfully on the effect of dutiful or negligent parents on their child's health, especially during those "dangerous summer" months. In these works, both Mom and Dad are depicted as potential sources of infection, but in all cases, the family's return to moral order either fittingly substitutes for—or, in the last example, successfully fends off—the (polio) threat to the child character's physical health.

Proto-Feminist Moments

Despite the paternalistic policies that shaped not only these magazines' response to polio but to world events and difficult subject matter of every kind, a broad range of likely unintentional textual effects may be seen to test, and thus testify to, women's ability to face serious social problems and examine (and expand) the limits of their individual spheres of influence. These effects indicate the proto-feminist subtext, however inadvertently mobilized, at work in these publications[79] and suggest the degree to which editorial attempts to shelter its readership were unwarranted and disserving. First it is worth noting the remarkably literate style characterizing almost all print media in this era, mainstream and women's publications alike. Browsing these volumes some fifty years after their release, one is struck by the sheer number of words —tiny-fonted ones—flowing in torrents over every oversized page. Even deodorant ads offered eight or 10 paragraphs of closely worded argument; news, features, fashion, and cooking were treated with the same elegant verbosity. *Good Housekeeping*'s "Memory Lane" and "Poetry Page" excerpted poems, quotes, speeches, and essays from the likes of Virgil, Houseman, and Churchill, while *Redbook* and *McCall's* presented "complete novels" in one or several issues.

Good Housekeeping's "Bureau" of research dominated the postwar issues, dividing its contents into Fashion, Beauty, Health, Children, and other sections, all of which were so detailed and even technical as to constitute a sort of advanced-degree curriculum in home management. Functioning as consumer advocate for an entire universe of women's commodities, each issue alerted women to advances in technology that transformed their appliances, fabrics, and cleaning products on an almost monthly basis. Reports from *Good Housekeeping*'s labs used a quirky lingo, coining terms (to accompany the newly minted technology) for the "densometer," which tested the water content in flour, the "shortometer," which measured shortening's various properties, and the "Fade-Ometer," which checked fabrics for colorfastness.[80] One infers from this striking verbal orientation an audience with broad powers of attention and concentration, large vocabularies, comfort with remote allusions, a willingness to learn while being entertained, and rapid reading abilities. These of course are the tools of the scholar and the intellectual, and it is remarkable that "ordinary housewives," whose cultural norms instilled an aptitude for language processing that astounds the modern reader, were considered then and are looked back on now as too unschooled and inept to deal straightforwardly with the crises of their day.

Additionally, these magazines told stories of financial and emotional hardship of real American women and their families, and depicted the home itself as a fertile medium for the readjustment of power structures regulating gender codes. While ultimately the novel roles these magazines offered readers are recouped by the sex-based imbalances of the period, new territory opens up nevertheless: in part, I argue, because fears of polio, the bomb, and communism caused fathers to turn to mothers for advice and strength and to share in the guilt and sorrow in times of frightening illness.[81]

The *Journal*'s semiregular feature "How America Lives" was a dependable source of hard-luck stories of struggling young marrieds or families of eight, whose meager home environments were depicted in minute detail and in the grim grays of black and white photography; the equally intrusive text examines the family's exhausting schedule, unmet debts, and budget shortfalls to the minute and penny. A *McCall's* article about *Strike It Rich*, "the radio program with a heart," recounts multiple hardship stories culled from the show,[82] and in a later issue the tragic details of eleven orphans' desperate circumstances are related.[83] We can assume female readers took compassionate interest in the tragic plights of these fellow-Americans or such fare would not have been a recurring feature. Thus women's interest in such narratives of personal disaster, and editors' willingness to open these worlds to their seemingly sheltered middle-class readership, make the diffident silence on polio, the most urgent family crisis of the era, a continuing curiosity.

Emily Martin has demonstrated the scientizing of housekeeping effected in these postwar publications in an effort to sanitize and thus immunize the home environment against polio and other invisible invaders.[84] Martin discusses the mania for cleaning and germ-fighting encouraged in homemakers during this period, thanks to the advances that had indeed come about in cleaning products and appliances and to the wealth of advertising that exhorted women to never be satisfied with less than utter spotlessness. While likely these pressures to eliminate invisible and potentially deadly germs from the home produced profound anxiety in mothers fearing the prospect of children sickened due to their "negligence" (about which more below), the scientized/technologized home environment positioned mother as chief scientist and the mastermind behind "germ warfare" in every home, empowering women in new ways and at last crediting her long hours spent behind a vacuum cleaner or dustrag, if not financially at least ideologically.

The breaking down of domestic spheres was also a raging design trend in this period, as kitchens opened onto living areas to create gender-mixed family spaces with only countertops and plant arrangements distinguishing mother's and father's traditional domains. The gender-blended zones of the backyard and barbecue grill were also regularly featured. Design plans provided the means to make the manly grill as kitchenlike as possible or to position the barbecue near the kitchen to coordinate food production activities.[85] By introducing topics of interest at the outermost rings of their readers' traditional environment, these publications enabled women to push at these boundaries literally and figuratively, to make gestures of kitchen- and home-leaving that might have been met with suspicion in more open contexts. In "She's Working *His* Way Through College" (*McCall's*), Yvonne is shown at work as a dental hygienist while Frank crouches on the floor to measure the evenness of her skirt hem;[86] in a short feature entitled "Mother Takes the Best

Pictures" (*McCall's*/Zeek), this traditional male role is conceded to women when it is recognized that "she's around when things happen that are worth photographing."[87] The story credits Mom with an eye for composition and a perspective on her children's personalities that is "better than any professional['s]."[88]

The *McCall's* "This is How I Keep House" series serves as an upbeat counterpart to the *Journal*'s sometimes-depressing "How America Lives" series. In both, the purpose is to introduce ordinary Americans to national readerships, examine their home life in almost intrusive detail, and provide a series of photographs of families in their intimate daily activities that provide their own line of fascinating commentary. Meanwhile, where the black-and-white photography of the "America Lives" series emphasized the families' downturning situations, "Keep House" insisted on cheery color photos of modern homes and families in the happy act of sharing chores or having fun. Yet if women were rushing through housework to have fun with the kids or relax with friends, were they endangering their family's well-being? How did the mother/homemaker balance her roles as lighthearted friend and activity coordinator to her children and no-nonsense dirt buster with little time for anything else?[89] A "Keep House" installment from a summer 1952 issue of *McCall's* — with, again, summer 1952 having the greatest number of polio infections in U.S. history—presents this striking mother's dilemma. On the surface of this story, homemaker Dorothy Hartley's play now/pay later philosophy is roundly endorsed by the text and attractively composed photos; the apologetics of this make-no-apologies credo must be located largely subtextually.

"Family fun comes first," breezes Dorothy in the epigraph to the story. "Work comes later," adds author Elizabeth Herbert approvingly.[90] The article describing this lifestyle vigorously supports Dorothy's family-first mentality—especially since the Hartleys live in a resort area of Massachusetts where outdoor life in the summer is especially pleasant— and congratulates her efficient, "no frills" approach to chores that "makes summer living pleasant for her family."[91] Herbert crows about the Hartleys' multiple time-saving appliances, especially the washing machine, and notes that on weekends even husband John is drawn into the fun as the family makes a day on his fishing boat. Yet despite the confidence exuded in these several remarks, elsewhere the article betrays a striking defensiveness of Dorothy's seemingly lax approach to homemaking, while the photo subject matter and captions undermine it almost entirely.

"Dorothy Hartley's reversal of housekeeping procedures in summer . . . does not imply poor homemaking," insists Herbert at one point. "Just the opposite."[92] Clearly, the need Herbert feels to fend off such criticism indicates its presence in the minds of her readership, who may look with suspicion on this shirking mother. In a later paragraph, Herbert's comment that "Dorothy doesn't believe in letting *every*thing slide in summer" recasts efficiency as "sliding" and rescues this lost sheep by assuring readers that even she has some scruples about home upkeep.[93] In fact, much of the article is at pains to describe how remarkably *busy* all five family members are—even when they are relaxing or having fun together—and the photos and captions do everything to reinforce this observation: only two of the ten depict the family *not* at work in the kitchen or on the boat.

So much for the play-first philosophy so proudly touted by mother and magazine in the headline of the piece. Even the most do-nothing of the photo compositions—mother and daughters relaxing on the Padanarum beach—is underlined by a reassuring list of their many activities: "While the three girls beachcomb, dig sand castles, swim, or sun, Dorothy camps in a sheltered cove, knits, mends, or reads."[94] Notably, this exposure to the beachfront is pointedly described as "health-giving" for the children; all three are pictured in long-sleeves or sweaters, and Dorothy avers that these outdoor excursions occur "while the day and the three little girls are cool, fresh."[95] Certainly, the coolness suggested by the words and images abates the threat supposedly carried by infectious diseases in the scorching heat of the summer months when bared bodies in close proximity spelled physical danger;[96] this woman's family, and her worthiness as a mother, are saved by the refreshing North Atlantic breezes that keep the deadly summer heat at bay twelve months a year.

Father Knows Best?

If women were enjoined, through stories like this, to shape up their housekeeping methods or face blame for a child's succumbing to unseen germs, on other occasions—especially those involving a child's long-term recovery from illness—they were urged to simply cede their authority to the necessary encroachments of their level-headed husbands. Such transfers of power are displayed frequently enough in these publications; either Dad is pictured taking control or Mother's ability to maintain her family's security and health—or even her own—is impugned by the magazines' hired authorities.[97] *Good Housekeeping*'s seemingly progressive regular features on "The Woman and Her Car" and "Woman and the Family Security" in fact raise questions as to women's ability to maintain family safety as often as they endorse her roles as independent driver and financial planner. While one "Car" installment suggests that women assume the role of driving the family on vacation[98] a later one called "Gadgets and Accessories" pictures a woman combing her hair in the mirror on the back of her sun visor.[99] Is this the kind of "gadget" one can use to fix a flat on the side of the road? And what is Mom doing in the driver's seat fussing with her hair? If she is acting responsibly and in fact saving hair care until she is sitting on the passenger side—the picture makes her position difficult to discern—she is evidently letting Dad drive after all; so much for "the woman and her car." One column in the "Security" series asks "What if *you* caused an accident?" and exhorts its accident-prone object of address to at least secure her family with adequate insurance policies.[100]

On the subject of children's health, a photo essay for *McCall's*, "Smitty Gets His Tonsils Out" (Smart)—and tonsillectomies during the summer months were considered as gateways to polio infection—pictures both Mom and Dad in hospital gowns, enacting the surgical moment at home, to prepare the youngster for his hospital stay.[101] In *Redbook*'s "Help Your Child GET WELL" (Taylor), both Mom and Dad observe the doctor put their boy's leg through a range of motion.[102] (Meanwhile, a photo caption reassures us that the problem is tuberculosis of the bone, i.e., not crippling polio.) Dad is positioned closer to the boy's head than is Mom and seen taking an active role in the boy's home recovery phase; the article cautions against *babying* a convalescing child—especially, as in the case here, a male child—and Dad is regarded as essential to avoiding this.[103]

In "The Convalescent Child" (*Good Housekeeping*/Kenyon) "Mother" is the primary referent—"If mother has had a home nursing course"; "a mother should ask the doctor"—seemingly granting wide authority to women on the serious occasion of a bed-bound child.[104] Yet such privilege is clearly a double-edged sword, as responsibility is conferred simultaneously with the suspicion that it will be mishandled. Inane questions such as "Is it easy for a mother to take care of a child during convalescence?" —of course the answer begins with "No"—and "Can a mother properly care for a convalescent child and also continue outside social activities?" insinuate that Mother is too weak-minded and/or self-absorbed to care for sick children without these heavy-handed prompts, so should perhaps not be given the job in the first place. In "Is Your Child Scared of the Doctor?" (*McCall's*/Baumgartner and Castle), Mother is pictured comforting her child before and after the traumatic "booster shot," while Dad is absent from the scene.[105] Yet if the title's questioning tone refrains from blaming Mom directly for her child's unhealthy fears, the article itself presents a series of strategies for helping the child overcome these fears, the ignoring of which will surely be on Mom's head. Her failure to adequately comfort, maintain a careful vigil, (conversely) avoid worrying, or follow doctor's orders is the subtext of many of these medical advice columns (i.e., "we wouldn't have to print these directives if women weren't so in need of them"), while the overriding tendency of inquiring mothers and responding doctors and editors to avoid questions about serious illnesses, especially polio, reveal these advisors — and position these mothers — as unqualified to handle the most difficult aspects of children's health.

The ground women gained in these several instances of the magazines' protofeminist gestures is decidedly lost when it comes to the issue of family health and safety. The texts discussed here concede women a certain sovereignty, only to immediately question women's ability with images of elaborately depicted disaster and a deluge of "advice" that exhorted, criticized, and offended their intelligence. Not surprisingly, the frightening situations (regarding polio, communism, and the atomic bomb) that so clouded present and future prospects for the postwar American family both opened the door on an interrogation of women's untapped strengths *and* indexed the anxiety that in the next moment triggered doubt in and denial of these strengths. Would that Evelyn R. Zeek, the author of "Mother Takes the Best Pictures," had been allowed to transfer the insights provided there to writings whose topics included home preservation, medical information-gathering, and child safety;[106] in addition to her camera work on a sunny afternoon, then, Mother would have been also credited with the presence (of mind and body), skillful hand, and careful eye that would have more than qualified her to guide children through doctor's visits and life-threatening illnesses and to receive information on both these subjects in her favorite women's publications.

Conclusion

As impossible as it would be to revisit the mindset of individual readers of these magazines during this period, the magazines themselves clearly demonstrate a fear of polio that manifested itself in remarkable ways. By offering at least occasional articles and fiction directly treating the subject, popular women's serials enabled women to contemplate one of their greatest fears, yet shaped each of these pieces around an inevitable happy ending that may have comforted some, maintained others in a state of dangerous denial, and perhaps deeply anguished those mothers whose own final chapters in the polio story had been anything but happy. These magazines' relentless positioning of women before (i.e., always at least one step ahead of) the polio crisis seems finally a function of their need to package the news, information, and even entertainment they produced as timely and useful, attributes meaningless to maternal readers for whom the magazine's mantra of affirming denial—not yet/not ever/not my child—came too late.

Aware of the dread and grief surrounding polio in the lives of their readers, these publications may have sought to provide the escapist fare that would heal wounds and generate higher sales figures, yet polio's pervasive presence in the maternal consciousness in this period likely "infected" many text elements touching on related themes—health, children, even water and summer—with its awful significance anyway. Yet the incipient feminism modeled, even inadvertently, in the many pages of these publications points toward a female readership remarkably equipped—intellectually, physically, and emotionally—to deal straightforwardly with life's most adverse conditions, indicating an ability to deal with more honest and effective discourse on polio that was largely unmet by their favorite leisure reading sources. This (untold) polio story is thus another example of the ideological context underestimating women's strengths, trafficking in the dissembling and silences that could even endanger lives and surely promoted ignorance, indifference, and isolation during a national health crisis.

2

"No Time for Tears"?: Gender, Fiction, and Denial in Polio Memoirs

IN CHARLES H. ANDREWS'S TELLINGLY TITLED *NO TIME FOR TEARS* (1951), ten-year-old Chuck (the author's elder son) succumbs to a serious polio infection, spending several days in the dreaded iron lung. His parents share feelings of impotence and desperation as they wait, in the hospital or at home, for signs of improvement, yet it is Andrews who takes the midnight call from the worried intern while wife Norma (who calls her husband "Daddy") "stand[s] beside me straining to hear." It is Norma who falls apart, while Andrews stoically insists she "take hold of [her]self";[1] Andrews's parents are summoned for support, and not surprisingly, it is Grandpa who takes charge, even ordering Norma to bed and organizing the younger kids for kitchen chores. After dinner he announces that "Mother [Grandma] will do the dishes and put the children to bed. Sonny and I will go to the hospital and call you from there."[2] Evidently, donning an apron and commandeering the kitchen posed little threat to Grandpa's ultimate authority to arrange Norma's access to her own sick child and take over, with his son, the role of intermediary in the all-important hospital setting.

When finally allowed to visit, Chuck's parents cheerfully invalidate his fear and sadness, and eventually the boy himself plays along, facing down a Halloween skeleton and joining his father in rating the nurses. When he learns that he may not go home for Christmas, he suffers an emotional setback, met by his parents with their typical wooden reaction: "He screwed up his face and began to cry again. . . . We remained immobile until he got control."[3] Following an indeed successful Christmas visit, Chuck returns to the hospital and is emotionally devastated.

In a climactic confrontation between Andrews and an imposing senior physician, paternal instinct butts against medical science—two modes of masculinity struggling for the right to "save" a little boy—and Andrews pulls his son from the hospital against medical advice. Luckily, Chuck suffers no setback from his early hospital release, although contemporary readers may cringe at the folly of a father's actions simply to appease his boy's emotional demands (earlier in the story, this would have been considered coddling) and salve his own wounded ego.

The parenting (i.e., fathering) methods depicted in this narrative reflect gender role conflicts and transformations elicited by the appearance of polio in the postwar American family, or at least nonfiction narratives about them. In the event of serious illness like polio, Mother's traditional role as temperature-taker and TLC-provider gave way to the encroachment of the house-calling doctor and the protocols of public health; Dad was the primary liaison with the public sector, but unless he himself had physician's credentials, he was reduced in the hospital setting to the roles of assistant, onlooker, or (much worse) obstruction or nuisance—roles usually ascribed to women and thus inherently threatening to men in these already emotionally fraught circumstances. Complicating the situation, ideologues as diverse as Freud and the anti-momist Philip Wylie had by now instilled in parents the sense that Mom's influence was ultimately poisonous to any child (especially any male child) beyond a certain age. To baby this older child was to (s)mother him or her; again, boys were thought especially endangered by this behavior, but in the wake of debilitating illness, when all children were called upon to be brave, tough, and resilient, boys' typical behaviors were foisted upon girls as well, and Dad's stern, unyielding manner was preferred for its therapeutic effects. The narrative indicates not only the pressure mothers surely felt to simply capitulate to their husbands' wishes, but also the threat fathers faced, who took over on these occasions only by stepping warily into Mother's shoes.

Certainly, this story would not have been written (by this author at any rate), had Chuck's near-total recovery not coincided so handily with his father's blustering philosophies about "ignoring handicaps."[4] Andrews credits his relentless bucking up with his son's recovery, while in fact Chuck may have done as well as he did *despite* his parents' emotional coldness and misguided doctoring, and with residual psychological damage nevertheless. Thus, Andrews's story illuminates not only the striking gender dynamics in play regarding saving a child from polio's permanent effects but also the role played by denial in polio nonfiction.

Before the specter of life-threatening disease, the stakes were radically raised in the playing out of traditional roles: when was it necessary to follow the rules or break subversively away from these in order to save the life of oneself or a loved one, and how did popular writings on this subject deal with such difficult questions? In narratives published in the postwar/polio period, was it manly to deny (ignore, surmount) the limitations polio may represent, or womanish to be in denial about (avoid, fear) these ultimately insurmountable limitations? In more recent accounts of polio survival, how have outdated gender divisions dissolved or simply reorganized themselves, and how do contemporary authors well versed in the politics of sex and gender bring their enlightened outlook to their discursive task? When does a polio memoir's use of fictional modes (embellishment, elision, digression, dialogue and scene fabrication) enlarge the function of denial in the work, and when does it productively complement an equally complex rendering of polio as "history"?

In what follows, I will consider polio nonfiction's gendered aspects ("masculine" versus "feminine" approaches), its readability as both fiction and history, and its status as text(s) in denial. This last will be a term of broad significance, as I question whether "strong" (i.e., masculine) or "weak" (i.e., feminine) writing is more in denial of polio's most troubling implications, how both the fictional and the historical may increase a memoir's debt to denial, and how both denial and depression are struggled through in various nonfiction accounts, on their way to healthy acceptance. For "how long do I keep trying?" is a necessary, difficult-to-answer question for every person recovering from polio and his or her medical team, who look to maximize muscle usefulness before terminating regular therapy sessions; who understand the importance of a determined, positive outlook; but whose optimism can shade suddenly and imperceptibly into an unhealthy state of denial that must be countered with a stringent "reality check." Conversely, too "realistic" an assessment can defeat a patient in the early recovery stages, can cripple with fear or depression before maximum recovery is achieved. Yet disability rights advocates have effectively questioned the social pressures placed on a weakened body to recover full potential when in fact only moderate recovery or total disability is in that body's range of abilities and long-term best interest. Where does one draw the line, therefore, between effort and acceptance? When does denial change from a vital coping strategy to an unhealthy mental state? Where lies that essential middle way between denial and depression, opposites that seem to cover the post-polio spectrum but are both in fact unhealthy responses that must be ultimately surmounted?

The shift from denial's intransitive form ("denying that") to its transitive form (to deny someone or something an intention or desire) has its own gender dynamic: often in polio writing, as well as in lived experience, who denies occupies a masculine position of power, while who is denied (deprived of) a voice, a presence, occupies the weakened, feminized position: the accused denies that he is guilty, yet the accusation itself puts the defendant on the defensive; the judge may deny the accused his freedom anyway. While impaired polio survivors are denied rights and access in an ableist culture on a daily basis—and are thus weakened, feminized, or desexualized in the process—it is also the case that polio memoirists may deny readers the entire story when they blithely insist they have denied polio a victory. Such a gesture is stereotypically strong, powerful, and masculine but belongs more correctly to the category of vulnerable, defensive maneuvering. Feminist disability theorists[5] critique the severance of discourse from bodily reality by reminding their readership that the personal (i.e., the bodily) is political; from a disability standpoint, then, "acceptance" refers not only to accounts of persons with polio coming to terms with their post-polio realities but also to those narrative moments that challenge ableist readers' most ingrained complacencies and force them toward total acceptance of the physically impaired in society.

Both acceptance and denial seem essential elements of the polio memoir, especially in the immediate postwar period. The primary point of publishing such a story was to cheer, instruct, and encourage readers facing the same crisis in their own families (or own bodies) or dreading the day when polio struck. If the women's magazines discussed in the preceding chapter positioned themselves (and thus perceived their readership) as permanently before polio, polio memoirs came clearly from within the polio experience and attempted almost always to pull the reader into this experience with specific details, a dramatic account, and/or emotional honesty. Conversely (though often, simultaneously), these memoirs moved toward the reader's own presumed state of ablebodiedness by doing all they could to put polio into the narrative past. For the polio-affected reader herself, the "inside story" of the polio experience was surely a space of affirming self-recognition, and the finally achieved states of physical or psychological recovery an invitation to join the author in polio's triumphant hereafter. Thus, while many with polio were drastically impaired (total paralysis, permanent iron lung usage) or even died from its complications, no one wrote (or was published) on this topic unless there was at least some good news to report.[6] In one remarkable account, six of seven children die inside iron lungs in one week.[7] Significantly, the narrator herself was the seventh child; such miraculous odds-beating was often the impetus for writing in the first place. Hugh Gregory Gallagher has pointed out that the "plot" of polio itself is upward-bound, encouraging further this optimistic trend: "Polio is not a progressive condition. Maximum paralysis occurs at the height of the critical stage of the disease; with informed exercise and care, over a period of months and years, the paralyzed muscles will regain—and *retain*—a significant degree of strength and function."[8]

Even in the contemporary period, when writers are much more inclined to present with honesty the worst of physical and emotional experiences generated by a life-changing illness, the pressure to produce what G. Thomas Couser has called "the comic plot expected of autobiography"[9] remains strong; the arrival at a serene and knowledgeable state of being may have occasioned, inspired, or enabled the writing in the first place. Who, after all, can create meaningful narrative from the depths of debilitating depression? Who has not at least found solace in the act of writing itself, which may lead the recoverer to new self-understanding and a sense of accomplishment simply by publishing the text? Writing itself, therefore, militates against the instance of the utterly hopeless story; even the surviving loved one, positioned to tell the tale of depression, debility, and death from polio, will incline toward the "meaningful message" as the story draws to a close or, again, why bother to write?[10] Finally this tendency may be chalked up to the middle-brow expectations of the audience toward whom these texts were and continue to be frequently aimed: moderate emotions, veiled allusions to sex and death, moral uplift.

Amy L. Fairchild suggests a division between "first-wave" and "second-wave" polio memoirs, locating a turning point in the mid-1950s, before which diffidence and optimism were the most common narrative modes and after which the women's, gay, and civil rights movements enabled (or required) illness biographers to confront the difficulty of their position from an equally radical perspective—with candor and graphic detail.[11] As accurate as this distinction is in many respects, I myself discern less a first and second wave than a spectrum of approaches to the subject, ranging between (rarely realized) endpoints of total acceptance and total denial. I suggest that, instead of a signal moment before and after which we recognize clear differences, traces of denial are present (sometimes pervasively) in even recently written texts, while some stories from the 1940s (the earliest decade I will consider here) break free from these constraints to shock and affect the reader. And if I read certain earlier texts as giving in thoroughly to denial, I also acknowledge that during these years, when polio remained a continuing threat and/or a pervasive source of sadness and concern, such attempts to soften harsh reality were a natural reaction and a necessary coping strategy. I also question whether the grim realities heaped upon the reader of more recent texts are to be preferred, simply because they open voyeuristically onto a disabled person's mental anguish, lost bowel control, and withered legs. The earlier texts are invaluable for what they convey to us about relations between genders and generations, well and sick roles of the period; and more recent offerings should not be read under any circumstances as having fully escaped the constraints of mainstream representation. Finally it will be difficult if not impossible to strictly separate those texts "in denial" from those texts "accepting of"; instead, elements of both denial and acceptance are widely locatable across the polio memoir canon and are most productively considered as the shifting, multivalent, pervasive phenomena that they are in the lived experience.

Critical Crossroads

Polio manifests as both an acute, sometimes life-threatening illness and, often, as a permanent, residual physical impairment of greater or lesser severity. My analysis of polio nonfiction thus intersects with two vital critical fields—literature and medicine studies and sociologically inflected disability studies, whose shared interest in the therapeutic aspects of the patient's own story is pertinent here. Their respective topics of inquiry, however, result in different core questions and shaping controversies: literature-medicine's focus on the narrative arc that is the illness experience itself (with its comic or tragic resolution in recovery or death) coincides well with literary analysts' (and ordinary readers') turn to literature for illumination of the universal human condition: as we are all sick at some point in our lives, fictional and nonfictional accounts of illness are in many ways the reader's own story. Readers embrace sick heroes and heroines, portrayed as complex characters in central roles; for literature-medicine theorists, patients and doctors in fiction and nonfiction—especially in contemporary writings—are most heroic when they function as partners, with patients taking an active role in their own recovery or, if necessary, end-of-life experience and doctors hearing and responding to their patients' points of view.

By contrast, the condition of physical or cognitive impairment and other bodily variations such as deformity or disfiguration is perceived by what Rosemarie Garland Thomson identifies as a "normate" readership (and its best-selling writers) with discomfort.[12] The misperception is that disability is an unnatural state of permanent suspension between sickness, recovery, and death; that only the rare individual finds him or herself in such unfortunate limbo; and that those who do are outside the human community in fundamental ways. "Normalcy narratives"[13] attempt to force disability into the illness-narrative paradigm, doing away with impairment through either miraculous recovery or the killing off of the affected character.[14] Thus disability theorists concern themselves with mainstream cultural representations that dehumanize and marginalize the impaired figure, that deny the commonplace reality of bodily non-normativity by making it into something alien and astounding.

True to their sociological origins, many disability theorists[15] analyze the collective response to (and responsibility for) impaired individuals, criticizing the tendency of the able-bodied mainstream to deny the reality, and the specific needs, of impaired fellow-citizens in myriad ways: failing to create a barrier-free society; refusing to accept physical limitation through worship of physical perfection and through relentless coaching of impaired loved ones to strive for full recovery; ignoring or discriminating against the physically impaired; and—most pertinent to this discussion—creating cultural representations that quarantine or minimize, or by contrast exaggerate and melodramatize, physical impairment. In Liz Crow's representative assessment, "dominant perceptions of impairment as personal tragedy are regularly used to undermine the work of the disabled people's movement and they rarely coincide with disabled people's understandings of their circumstances. They are individualistic approaches."[16] Also Lennard J. Davis: "by narrativizing an impairment, one tends to sentimentalize it, and link it to the bourgeois sensibility of individualism and the drama of the individual story."[17] In these critiques, "the individual" or "the personal" names and invalidates both the physical body and the narrative depicting its illness or impairment experience.

Yet this intense—and persuasive—antinarrative bent is balanced by the work of others in disability studies who allow that individual accounts do benefit both writers and readers, impaired and normate. Distinguishing between the socially created, ideologically supported phenomenon of disability and the personalized, physical, cognitive, and emotional reality of bodily impairment, these writers argue for a balancing and integration of the social and personal, the discursive and the physical, rejecting the stringent anti-individualist, disability-only orientation of social-model theorists. Impairment studies practitioners, if you will, come often from a feminist perspective and divide the impairment/disability focus between female and male disability theorists.[18] A crystallizing example is Margrit Shildrick and Janet Price's questioning of Michael Oliver's influential pronouncement that "disablement is nothing to do with the body."[19] Corker and French argue for the interrelation of disability and impairment experiences and note "the role of [individual] discourse in creating *and challenging* disability oppression."[20] Implicitly, these theorists argue that attempts to deny the impaired body its meaning and importance resemble the denial suffered at the hands of the able-bodied mainstream.

Thus theorists of impairment share the pronarrative stance of literature-medicine experts, who embrace the empowering qualities of illness narrative. Yet the discussion that follows is informed by all three approaches: social-model theory underwrites my critique of denial (even self-denial) in polio memoirs, feminist-oriented "impairment studies" informs my discussion of gender stereotypes and the special issue of women with impairments, while literature-medicine theory reinforces my contention that progressive, therapeutic, personalized responses to the polio experience indeed exist and are as worthwhile to preserve and interpret as are narratives that tend finally to perpetuate prejudice and misunderstanding.

Literature-medicine theorists explore the illness narrative's frequent departure from the realistic account. Recurrent is the emphasis on plot,[21] for example Chambers and Montgomery's reference to the "shaping power"[22] of illness narrative plotlines and Cheryl Mattingly's description of the benefits of "therapeutic emplotment."[23] For Mattingly, "the exaggeration, play, and love of the fantastic so often found in ritual, myth, and folktale . . . is evidently particularly suited to our very human need to understand and cope with the very real things that happen to us."[24] To presume the stories we tell about our illnesses will mirror accurately our lived experiences of these is to indulge in a "naive realism" critiqued in her work.[25] Arthur Kleinman agrees that "myth making . . . reassures us that resources conform to our desires rather than to actual descriptions," and that "self-deception makes chronic illness tolerable."[26] Finally, Arthur Frank contends that even "evasive" personal narratives cannot be dismissed as false testimony: "I have read personal accounts I considered evasive, but that evasion *was* their truth."[27]

Yet later in his argument, Frank posits that the narrator of his own illness "rises to the occasion . . . by telling not just any story but a good story,"[28] and that "the good story refuses denial."[29] While Frank spoke favorably of the "evasive" story a moment ago, here he comes out against "denial" in favor of this striking cultural phenomenon, the "good story." For each of the three perspectives examined here, this term has its own meaning: social-model theorists might use the term ironically to refer to a sentimentalized or overdramatized account that allows the reader a good cry and a happy ending; for them, the only good story is no story. Impairment studies specialists and literature-medicine theorists might take the same emotion-laden narrative and assign it a positive value, or—as above, celebrate stories that escape heavy emotion through fantasy, ritual, and evasion. I believe, however, that when Frank calls for good stories, he searches out well-told tales that touch upon significant human truths, that confront their situations honestly, recognize (not necessarily surmount) limitation, and set the reader firmly in the author's (or biographical subject's) shoes—or respirator, as the case may be.

I consider this kind of account to be a "strong" story, whether written by or about a man or woman, and throughout this essay will question gender assumptions that equate strength with masculinity and with "beating polio." While many among the polio-affected made full recoveries, many faced harrowing periods of illness and rehabilitation on the way to their final post-polio state. The truly carefree encounter with polio (many had minor infections) would not have been published; therefore, polio narratives, almost by definition, emerge from a traumatic illness or permanent impairment and deal with this trauma in striking ways. The phenomenon of denial in these narratives enables us to examine the function of "strength," "victory," the happy ending, and idealized forms of masculinity and femininity in postwar and contemporary polio texts.

Failed Fathering

At the start of this chapter, I considered how a polio father, validated by his acquiescing wife, may or may not have emotionally (and even physically) damaged his son by pushing relentlessly for full recovery. Andrews's *No Time for Tears* is an invaluable account of parenting in an era of tough love; his and his wife's emotional coldness are enacted to avoid the "self-pity and neuroticism"[30]—that is, the sissification and permanent disability—of a male child affected by polio. Modern-day accounts by polio survivors continue to single out Father as the parent whose various ways of denying the problem did more harm than good. Ironically, despite the notion circulated in the polio period, that Father's firm methods were essential to a child's recovery from serious illness, adult polio survivors report the opposite to be the case.

Mary Grimley Mason's father was evidently a classic example of the polio parent who refused to give up. Significantly, both parents were absent from the home—father on business overseas, mother traveling to meet him for vacation—when Mason came down with the virus in 1932. Mason's father returned in record time from Japan to Philadelphia, where Mason was hospitalized,[31] and must have been plagued by numerous unanswerable questions: had his child taken sick because he left her for such a distant destination? because he had allowed his wife to be gone from the house during the same period? Had she survived the potentially deadly attack because he had gotten back "in time"? In what other ways would his daughter's prognosis depend upon his future actions? In the child's convalescent phase, it is the high-level occupation, which removed her father from the family post in the first place, that provides the financial means to explore every therapeutic avenue—long after his daughter's body has reached its recovery limit.

Mason's father gets second opinions from countless specialists, explores a nerve-crushing therapy to no avail,[32] and insists his daughter attempt ambulation with less obtrusive canes instead of her mobility-enhancing crutches. He verges on the physically abusive, even striking his wife during an argument once and raising a hand to Mason herself. While her father dies in a drowning accident while she is still a young girl—three days after he almost strikes her, in fact—Mason is haunted by his dispiriting disappointment in her all her life. Waiting for his body to be recovered, she—entirely appropriately—feels no guilt for her part in their final argument or, as is conceivable, for causing her father to drown, but only "that I have not grieved for his death."[33]

Psychologist Garrett Oppenheim deals remarkably with his life-long perception that he (or his disability) *is* to blame for the departure from the family of his biological father and, strikingly, for the death by heart attack of his beloved stepfather. Compounding the guilt feelings of many children-of-divorce is the disabled child's sense that his physical limitations are the result of former misbehavior, that he himself is bad or defective, and thus to blame for his parents' problems. The guilt feelings in Oppenheim's case are all but confirmed by his biological father, a renowned poet whose *Mystic Warrior* actually recounts the moment of his son's succumbing to polio as the "symbol of his ruined marriage."[34] Later in life, during an interval of stress at work, his stepfather, a physician, "climb[s] four flights of stairs"[35] to treat a family friend at young Oppenheim's behest. The friend has only a bad cold, and the anger his stepfather displays upon his return home initiates a bout of chest pains that results in his death three days later. Though Oppenheim "race[d] through the streets as fast as [his] brace and cane would take [him]"[36] to obtain the heart medicine that in fact postponed his father's demise, he blames himself for the crisis, and indeed the boy was tragically if only tangentially implicated in his stepfather's death.

Despite the striking temporal parallels in the stories of Mason's and Oppenheim's fathers' deaths, the children's reactions could not be more different. Mason's physical, emotional, and moral innocence frees her from feelings of responsibility, yet the inability to mourn her father's loss, effected by his loveless treatment of her, grows into an emotional "disability" that follow her throughout life (see discussion below). Where Mason's father refuses to give up on her rehabilitation, Oppenheim's father does not even try, eliciting the deep emotional turmoil in his son that is exacerbated by the death of his devoted second father. Meanwhile, Mason's freedom from guilt is the state toward which Oppenheim must work; clearly his stepfather's heart was about to give out at any rate, and his feelings of responsibility for this father's death are likely an after-effect of his first father's rejection. Despite the early death (or departure) of all three fathers, then, both authors suffer life-long emotional upheaval because of them, a form of emotional paralysis—i.e., pain that will not start (in Mason's case) or stop (in Oppenheim's)—that only worsens their impaired physical situation.

The father depicted in Robert Huse's story resembles and departs from the fathers already discussed. He remained with the family but withdrew emotionally from his polio-affected son; as opposed to the financial reserves that enabled Mason's father to pursue multiple therapeutic options, even during the Depression, the Depression-era finances of Huse's family are no match for the seaside rehabilitation Huse's mother plans. The family does not even own a car for the trip, and his father must struggle to cover his son's expenses, with growing resentment toward the boy and his ever-"optimistic" mother. In the family's escalating Freudian drama, Huse's mother directs not only all of the family's income but also her time and energy to the recovery of her son; after hiring a maid to free up more of his wife's time for "his needs," Huse's father realizes with exasperation that the maid "simply meant that [his wife] was able to spend more time with [her son]. She read aloud to [him] more and [they] drew even closer together."[37]

One winter, Huse's father takes the boy sledding and pushes him into a tree. The "accident" results in only a sprained ankle, but this is surely a serious enough setback for a boy already requiring crutches. While his father leaves no ultimate physical scar, Huse, like Mason and Oppenheim, is lastingly affected by his father's emotional abuse, indicating that his own situation as a "father and husband facing marital problems later in life"[38] is a result. While Huse's father is certainly right to resent exclusion by his own family, it is clear that the problem is not the boy himself but his own inability to assert his prerogative (Huse's word is "inhibited") and his mother's suffocating "optimism" (i.e., denial). Thus Huse's father's "unreasoning wrath"[39] is clearly misdirected, and the genre of polio nonfiction adds another story of a child hobbled by a father's rejection to its lists.[40]

The most abusive father in this survey is Anne Finger's mentally unbalanced family tyrant, depicted in moving detail in *Elegy for a Disease* (2006). In chapter 3, I will discuss Finger's novel, *Bone Truth*, about a polio-affected young woman whose impairment during girlhood is only one of many problems — and nowhere near the largest one — faced by her chaotic, ultra-leftist family. In Finger's own life, her polio-related impairment does not keep her from climbing stairs at school and at home, and is indeed a minor incident compared to the trauma and upheaval caused by her sexually harassing, heavy-drinking, all-around abusive father. While he humiliates and harangues all four of his children, it is primarily his polio-affected daughter whom he goes after physically, choking her on several occasions, causing her to black out and nearly suffocate. In terms that resonate across this discussion, "His anger toward me was physical, rage at that body of mine that persisted, despite all the promises that had been made to us, despite all that had been done for it, despite all that had been done to it, in remaining crippled. His daughter's body — and for him the operative word was 'his'. . . . Out there for all the world to see, the physical manifestation of the inner state of our family — broken, bent, crippled, wrong."[41] It is perhaps the father's societally instilled sense of ownership of his family's bodies and futures that elicited these damaging paternal reactions to polio onset in the postwar context. Certain fathers felt threatened and betrayed by their children's "failure" to surmount polio and pushed physically and emotionally to solve the problem, despite the ultimate impossibility of doing so.

Male Polio Patients

Turnley Walker's *Rise Up and Walk* (1950) complements Charles Andrews's story, depicting a man of Andrews's temperament and outlook as the patient instead of the father. Like Andrews's, Walker's narrative style is blithe and quick-paced. Short, "muscular" sentences and a jazzy, Runyonesque patter characterize both stories, and both authors use humor to entertain their readers and inspire those who are dealing too fretfully with polio—in Andrews's case his son, in Walker's the guy in the next bed. Daniel J. Wilson notes that the "anxieties about work"[42] expressed in Walker's narrative indicate the crisis in masculinity polio represented, yet I read the fixation on work/finances as the "manly response," supplanting fears regarding one's emotional, physical, and sexual status: Walker's "delirium" causes him to forget the revisions of a novel he wants to write, and he dwells anxiously not on lost mobility or bladder function but lost business as a PR executive. Despite the anxieties felt by the narrator regarding residual weakness, inability to provide for his family, and so on, he leaves the hospital under his own ambulatory steam; as they near their release dates, Walker and his fellow-patients "yell with laughter" and "make crazy, happy gestures with their fists,"[43] and the "victory" enjoyed on the final page is for health and masculinity, which, for this male author and many among his original readership, are one and the same.

Wilson considers the particular shade of crisis polio represented to men, who labored under mid-century social mandates to function as winners in sports and other physical contests, sole breadwinners, stoic authority figures, and shapers of a married couple's sexual relationship. He notes that "the popular name, infantile paralysis, itself illustrates the challenge the disease posed to masculinity," in that polio "created an infant-like dependency"[44] in supposedly rugged men. Meanwhile, Wilson quotes Leonard J. Kriegel who writes of having "beaten" and "overcome" polio[45] as signs of this successful compensation, while below I will question whether such stereotypically masculine terminology is not indicative of yet more anxiety and uncertainty.

Here as well it helps to reintroduce Fairchild, whose findings corroborate an observation made by Kriegel with respect to polio, that "Simply put, a woman endured whereas a man fought back."[46] In the contemporary narratives that are her primary focus, this distinction largely holds, and while I will consider the issue of the woman's narrative response to polio below, I observe here that the concept of "fighting back" contains multiple and contradictory gender associations. Certainly, the men punching their fists in the air of Walker's narrative suggest the sort of hypermasculine battle with illness indicated in Kriegel's formulation, but in this same traditional context, the idea of "kicking up a fuss," complaining about service, or fighting for patients' rights and wheelchair accessibility must be seen as irrelevant to a "real man's" focus on rapid release from the hospital and complete recovery. In fact the supreme stoicism sought after in, for instance, Andrews's demand that his wife "get a hold of herself," resembles the "endurance" ascribed by Fairchild to stereotypically female narratives; while patience, silence, and acquiescence are certainly attached to a feminized concept of the term, in fact both enduring and fighting back lend themselves to masculine *and* feminine stereotypes. I myself find the most typically masculine tendencies among these narratives (many of them written by women) to substitute issues related to fighting (high emotion, "struggle," "desperation") with clear-cut victories, as the patient-protagonist moves confidently from one goal to the next, and little if any time is spent contemplating the valleys between the peaks. By contrast, fighting connotes the noisy, outlandish reactions of authors like Lorenzo Wilson Milam, whose "bad attitude" toward careless nurses and condescending well-wishers may be regarded as a model of patient rights advocacy but suggests just as well the "bitchy" personality attributed to certain gay men whose effeminacy removes them from traditional masculine categories.

While Milam writes remarkably of the double burden of homosexuality and polio-related disability in an era before the mainstream dealt decently with either, the conflicted masculinity displayed (almost entirely inadvertently) by Bentz Plagemann telling his story several decades earlier suggests yet another means by which traditional notions of manhood were threatened by the adult onset of polio. In *My Place to Stand* (1949), Plagemann tells the story of his literal failure to fight, of his falling ill with polio mere days before his naval hospital ship was supposed to join a WWII battle off the coast of France, and the crisis of masculinity set off—in himself and his fellow-sailors—by his "shirking." Certainly the unfortunate timing is compounded by what was undoubtedly Plagemann's sensitive, effete presence among the uncouth, rough-and-tumble sailors he served with. A serious, even (by his own account) humorless, poetic type who inclines toward fussy, Romantic phrasings like "our hearts quickened" and "excited the admiration of his fellow-sailors," Plagemann is a pharmacist's assistant on board his ship, who takes Whitman (of all people) as a wartime role model and faints at the sight of blood. Such scandalous weakness is duly noted in stories that run like wildfire around the ship, though the taunts of "sissy" and "pansy" Plagemann likely suffered at the hands of his compatriots are not recorded in the narrative.

In fact, Plagemann takes every opportunity to signify his heterosexual status, starting with a reference to his wife in the opening line and likening his blood-queasiness to that of his hypermasculine grandfather, who "fathered a large family and could endure [note the verb choice] great personal hardships without complaint"[47] but who, alas, had to kill the Sunday chicken with his eyes closed. During his treatment for and recovery from polio, Plagemann's fidgeting in bed,[48] frequent complaints against the military hospitals he recovers in, and intense shyness with his fellow-convalescents at Warm Springs[49] are behaviors perfectly acceptable for anyone in Plagemann's situation, but following the lengthy, defensive, and revelatory introduction, these behaviors seem like so much "fussing" and distinctly counter to the real man's approach.

Leonard Kriegel is a contemporary author dealing more forthrightly with the issue of masculinity threatened by polio. In *Flying Solo* (1998) he offers provocative chapter titles such as "Bodily Passions: Hephaestus among the Gods" and "Pursuing Women, Meeting Myself," and interrogates the mid-century mania (hardly outgrown today) with "being a man," conceding that "such clichés spring from the culture that give them life, and to the idea of what it meant to be a man in 1944 I owe my survival."[50] As a writer, Kriegel attends to the thrust of words and analyzes related terms—manly, manhood, to be a man. Meanwhile, and despite Fairchild's crediting him as "the most influential of [contemporary polio] writers,"[51] his text is reminiscent of Plagemann's reticent narrative from fifty years earlier; specifically, both take interest in post-polio heterosexual masculinity, yet weaken the effort with writing by turns vague, overwrought, and banal. While Kriegel frankly approaches the issue of disability sexuality, asking "How did a cripple fuck?"[52] he never provides the answer to this question. Throughout, he sacrifices what is most meaningful about his conflicted relationships to women (and the world) for trite or obscure formulations.[53] Finally, Kriegel's provocative question regarding how "cripples fuck" is answered only with a much more general question: "What is it that we want from women?"[54] Using generalized terms such as "we" and "one," Kriegel shifts the context from his particular situation to that of men in general. While he has every right to consider himself an ordinary man dealing in ordinary ways with the "mars/venus" dilemma, his impairment-oriented inquiry disappears as he does.

More curious is this book's tendency to overstate a polio memory in such a way as to threaten its plausibility. In the early days of rehabilitation, Kriegel and his fellow-patients quake in fear of warm water hydrotherapy, a method of treatment described as pleasant and beneficial by polio patients since Roosevelt. Later he overreacts in extreme fashion when his wheelchair is delivered—"I wanted to shout with joy for a happiness that was a jubilant, most unmechanical gift. I wanted to bellow my liberation for the entire ward to hear."[55] In fact he "loved that wheelchair with a passion that embarrasses [him] to this day,"[56] yet pages later "refused to think about a wheelchair as an alternative to walking on crutches and braces. In fact I avoided thinking about wheelchairs at all."[57] In an epiphanic moment from his youth, "anger" simultaneously "hurled me into my fear" and "purged me of my terror."[58] Later he is returned to his wheelchair by the medically impossible diagnosis of "the broken femur of my right hip, the carpal-tunnel syndrome of my left elbow."[59] So improbable are these dramatic reversals that the experience seems to have come by vicariously, until the reader is forced to question whether Kriegel had polio at all. This question is entirely rhetorical—Kriegel is certainly a polio survivor—but the writing itself obscures his experience.

Declining to put up a brave front are two accounts of men's polio experience bravely located in the agonized, transforming body itself. In the opening chapters of *Black Bird Fly Away* (1998) Hugh Gregory Gallagher suffers alone in confusion and misery, spending an entire night under pounding hot water in the shower of his college dormitory, the only therapy that eases his searing pain.[60] In the hospital he clings to life by a thread, surviving total paralysis and iron lung support when he promises his mother that he will live instead of give up.[61] On a fateful night following release from the iron lung, an "older cranky nurse" forcibly disimpacts him, a gesture of violation that Gallagher equates with "rape" and blames for "problems with sexuality and problems with authority, which I have yet to resolve satisfactorily."[62] In later chapters, Gallagher deals frankly with the complications from this incident, both a lifelong struggle with severe constipation and psychosexual inhibitions.

Jim Marugg's *Beyond Endurance* (1954) is a woman-authored text—Ann Walters receives top credit, although it is written in Marugg's own first-person—that likewise deals in gripping detail with the horror of polio in its early stages, including high fever, confusion, and nightmarish hallucinations.[63] It moves almost subconsciously from the narrator's state of mind to his nether regions, specifically his reproductive organs and threatened manhood. As opposed to the professional and financial concerns dwelt upon in, for instance, Walker's narrative, Marugg describes the specifically sexual threat posed by polio. In a fever, he dreams that "they had taken my body apart in the night and I couldn't find the pieces. I began to search wildly. Among the tumbled blankets. Under the bed. In the chest among my shirts and underwear. In the closet. In the bathroom."[64] The loaded references to the bed, bathroom, and underwear indicate the "pieces" the narrator is most desperate to recover, while "the closet" connotes the shame produced by the prospect of an unmanned life.

Later, Marugg imagines himself as a corpse autopsied by medical students, one of whom immediately "points with a scalpel" to the "reproductive organs";[65] in another dream he "had been castrated!"[66] In more lucid moments, he worries that his best friend, who drives his wife to the hospital, is threatening his marriage; a triumphant scene later returns Marugg to the "driver's seat" when he obtains a car with hand controls. Beyond these several references to threatened gender/sexual function Marugg treats the agonies of severe bulbospinal infection and the arduous recovery process with brutal honesty. Such forthright accounts demonstrate courage and strength, ensuring the intact masculinity of a male narrator, despite (or perhaps due to) his honestly expressed sexual anxieties, much more effectively than do transparent efforts to put up an impervious front. I am less inclined to credit his female ghostwriter with the qualities of this account than to regard it as no coincidence that Marugg is comfortable enough to both entrust a woman with the presentation of his story and share so openly what frightens him most about his polio experience.

Above I implied a critique of a simplistic equation between masculinity and total health, and here I am equally intent to avoid suggesting that because Walker's, Plagemann's and Kriegel's treatments of their subject are vague, circular, and misleading they are in any way "gay." Of the male authors considered here, only Milam comes out explicitly as a gay man. The more flexible concept of "conflicted masculinity" helps us to read a range of traditional and unorthodox male behaviors in relation to disability and authorial styling: significantly, both hyper- and hypo-masculine textual displays are *equally* capable of denying polio's true pains and sorrows; finally, I suggest that weakened male bodies reverse their situation most effectively by writing "strong" stories (such as Gallagher's and Marugg's) about their polio experience and recovery—stylistically proficient, thematically honest, psychosexually undefended.

Women and Polio

Women authors of polio narratives are not immune to the self-protective maneuverings around difficult issues so commonly attributed to the fragile egos of men, and the range of subject positions adopted by the authors discussed here with respect to gender, sexuality, and disability are as varied and instructive as those of the male narratives. An important distinction, however, regards women's versus men's approach to the subject of sexuality; as Fairchild notes, women authors tend to be even more reticent on the subject of physical relations,[67] and none of the authors considered here "comes out" in her narrative as anything other than traditionally heterosexual. Sexuality, therefore, implies the narrower notion of heterosexuality, narrowed further still to the prospects of marriage or divorce but opening into the important issue of spousal relations and the ability to bear and maintain custody of children following polio. Thus a sexual politics of polio-related disability emerges in each case, even if these are extremely conservative politics, even if they are never outlined as such directly.

Eleanor Chappell's biography of Bea Wright, a mid-level executive with the March of Dimes, who herself became infected with polio shortly before taking on this role, can be safely regarded as the most in-denial of all the women's texts discussed here—if not the most in-denial in the entire survey. So bound is this author to the conventions of ladylikeness that polio appears here primarily as an unspeakably shameful secret. In fact, Wright's illness is multi-pronged and life-threatening, and her recovery process was evidently as lengthy and arduous as was anyone's return from total paralysis; in addition, her pre-polio life, as a divorced mother of three children, surely had its trials that might have been depicted honestly, but Chappell is determined instead to whitewash these difficulties with every stroke. Somehow she has managed to make Wright's life-changing experience almost boring; again, the relatively recent date of this publication (1960) indicates the tenacity of the gender roles shaping these polio narratives.

Everyone, including Helen Hayes who writes the foreword to this book, is struck by Wright's remarkable beauty, and this pretty lady's story of an ugly disease turns almost immediately to her alarming symptoms. The classic fever and stiff neck have Bea worried, but work, sons (even named Tom, Dick, and Harris), and a string of admiring beaux call her back to life, and she proceeds gracefully around her illness for several days. Note the blend of trouble, glamour, even eros in the following passage:

> Taking a deep breath, she crossed to the closet and picked out a crisp white linen suit to wear.
> Casting a longing look at the bed, rumpled from a night of broken sleep, she put on a pair of sheer hose, amazed that the soft brush of the nylon hurt her legs.
> As she slipped into the linen suit, the material hurt her body where it rubbed against it, and the pain in her head strove to blot out reason. Pulling on a pair of gloves with shaking hands, she began to review the agenda for the day. . . .
> As she started down the apartment stairs to catch a bus, for no apparent reason, she fell. Lying at the bottom of the stairs, the freshness of her white suit ruined, Bea looked about in bewilderment. What had happened? She got up slowly, went back to her room, changed clothes, then started out again — more carefully this time.[68]

Pathos gathers inadvertently throughout this account, as the reader fears for this sweet, lovely lady, so addled by clothes-consciousness and her busy agenda that she risks life and limb before summoning the necessary assistance. If Mother always said to wear clean underwear in case one wound up in the hospital, Bea will evidently make sure that she greets her medical team with an entire knockout ensemble.

Once hospitalized, Bea is diagnosed with bulbospinal polio (a one-two punch of breathing restriction and limb paralysis) and endures a high fever and painful muscle spasms. Chappell refers to "unbearable pain"[69] but does nothing to actually depict this; in two paragraphs we are whisked from diagnosis to rehabilitation,[70] and this devastating episode is minimized into meaninglessness. Instead, Chappell generates interest and sympathy from the sea of children surrounding Bea in the emergency room and hospital ward. She comforts Jimmy who is afraid and missing his mother,[71] and Larry, "who smiled all day . . . and cried bitterly at night when the lights were turned out"[72]; she even volunteers as story-reader and substitute mother in the children's ward as soon as she is up in a wheelchair.

Significantly, the suffering of her own children due to her situation is downplayed. Tommy, the youngest, is "sent to Wisconsin to stay with relatives"[73] for an unspecified duration, while the two older boys remain home on their own until Mother is well. In fact, Bea returns to health, makes a trip to DC, and enjoys several dinner dances with various admirers before reuniting, in the progress of the narrative at any rate, with her youngest son. On a compensating trip to Europe, Tommy is cheerful and graciously interested in Bea's millionaire husband-to-be, yet the loss, rejection, and insecurity this child surely dealt with during his mother's health crisis is ignored. Even Bea herself is a sympathy-deserving child of a mother who writes a "cold and unemotional" letter[74] acknowledging Bea's illness, yet Chappell forbids Bea to react sadly on this occasion. Instead she plays out an emotionally robust reunion with her mother—once she has largely recovered—later in the story.[75] In Chappell's effort to ensure the reader that no one need pity Wright in her situation, she limits her reader's ability to care about her at all. Appropriately, Wright's is probably the most total recovery of any of the polio protagonists' considered here. In her foreword, Hayes watches her "walking, firmly and gracefully, looking completely lovely"[76] at her son's graduation, reassuring the reader before the story even begins that a thoroughly happy ending is in store.

Forty years later, Mary Grimley Mason's *Life Prints* (2000) departs from and converges with its precursor in striking ways. Clearly Mason is the more skilled writer; while Chappell labored to tell a pretty story, Mason's style seems effortlessly beautiful, though its smoothness and understatement may do more to block our access to her story's harsh realities than open onto them. On multiple occasions in this narrative, Mason recognizes her "denial" regarding disability, yet does not seem to move past this state in her writing. The quietude of the prose makes this plain; in painful moments she speaks of "rejection"[77] and "devastation"[78] but is in total control as she relives these emotions. She is a surprisingly fretful child during recovery at Warm Springs, taking offense at having to hold a string on a turkey ("I was no one's poster child") and sitting next to FDR at Thanksgiving dinner. This willful attitude, however, gives way to the roles of "drifting" academic and "supportive" spouse, and the reader is struck by her equanimity in the face of permanent limitation and destructive interpersonal relationships (especially with her husband).

Indeed, Mason's impairment seems to have been relatively minor, with the cloud on her horizon her disappointing husband instead. Clearly, she supports this dilettante through years of briefly held jobs, unfinished manuscripts, and halfhearted courses of study; despite her less than total physical strength and the added responsibilities of three children to bear and raise, it is she who brings in most of the family income, while Herb deals with depression and alcoholism and initiates several affairs. Mason notes these bad behaviors but never complains about them; expressing "discontent" and "frustration" with teaching secondary school to earn Herb's keep,[79] she nevertheless accompanies him to France, where she must again earn the income while he enjoys a zealous conversion to Catholicism, and trade in her hand-controlled car for total dependence on Herb and his Renault. If Mason's physical situation is successfully denied, she is instead in denial about the dismal state of her marriage, and Fairchild has pointed to the issue of disabled women being abused or left behind by marital partners, much more often than are men;[80] in her narrative, Mason inhabits the role of a woman whose self-esteem is weakened by her disability and who is thus willing to tolerate an exploitative marriage. It is a relief when she is finally freed of this man, yet it is he who leaves the marriage when Mason should have thrown him out, or at least transcribed into her autobiography the writing visible on the wall, years earlier.[81]

In contrast to Chappell/Wright's and Mason's narratives, which deny the ramifications of impairment (for Chappell/Wright physically, for Mason emotionally) in such remarkable ways, Noreen Lidunska's early memoir, *My Polio Past* (1947), presents its reader with the intensities of polio onset in graphic detail. While her flippant tone departs from the reserved stylings of both Chappell and Mason, recalling the irreverent posturings of Andrews and Walker instead, the humor clashes with but does not obscure the depths of physical suffering she depicts and obviously endured. All of these women "walk away" from their polio pasts; Chappell/Wright by treating the illness/recovery episode as briefly as possible, Mason by confining much of her polio-related narration to the early chapters, renewing our sense of polio as a "child's disease." While Lidunska also moves past acute illness to rehabilitation and continuous improvement, her early chapters, depicting her infection/illness episode, are the most memorable of the book. Describing her throat paralysis, "The water just stayed in my throat, until it began to trickle in a thousand and one wrong directions. My larynx helped make horrible noises, and I leapt out of bed, drowning."[82] Later, it was "as though an arrow-borne match had been shot into a stack of dried leaves, I felt a tremor in my lower back, and the bonfire ignited."[83] Lidunska's ladylike aplomb and sprightly metaphors do nothing to mitigate the pain she depicts here; almost in spite of herself, she has created a singularly arresting picture of polio for a woman author (for any author, in fact) of this period.

Fairchild applauds this text for its portrayal of the defiant patient. In her rehabilitation phase, Lidunska refuses to make a stuffed teddy bear at the behest of her occupational therapist, and Fairchild contrasts such "rebels" with the damaging image of the "good patient."[84] Meanwhile, we return here to the interesting double-sidedness of concepts like "fighting" and "rebellion": the patient's cheeky attitude with the hospital staff coincides with the author's swaggering tone, yet like Andrews and Walker before her, these only work narratively speaking since Lidunska was lucky enough to have done it "her way" (i.e., ignoring her therapist's instructions) and still gotten to leave the hospital without crutches. For myself, this text's main offering is less its rebel protagonist than its shocking opening moments. While the story moves from the pit of dire illness to almost total recovery, this pit is not skimmed or hung with lace curtains but bravely, graphically dwelt in.

Gender and Sexuality in the Iron Lung

Very likely, the fullness of recovery enjoyed by the polio survivor/protagonist, or the limitation of involvement in the first place, contributes in significant ways to a polio memoirist's tendency toward denial, understatement, and traditionally gendered approaches to life and writing: reserve for female authors, swaggering for men. The less permanent or noticeable the residual impairments for any polio-affected woman, for instance, the more likely she was to win herself a husband and, in the 1950s and 1960s when these women would have been marrying, the more likely she would be to adapt a traditional woman's outlook on women's roles, illness and disability, and the choices one makes when writing for publication. Tragically, it is perhaps the severity of impairment that we can in part thank for the radical approaches to women's roles and polio writing on display in two very different women-authored texts, Jane Boyle Needham's *Looking Up* (1959) and Kathryn Black's *In the Shadow of Polio* (1996). Needham herself and Black's mother Virginia never progressed beyond the rocking bed (a seesawing mattress that mimics the push-pull breathing assistance of the iron lung); while Needham is still alive and metaphorically kicking at the end of her narrative, Black's mother dies after two years of physical and emotional confinement, and from each of these outcomes emerges each narrative's remarkable contribution to the discussion of disabled women's rights. In this same genre, several male-authored stories of permanent, polio-induced respirator requirement break the most rules with respect to men discussing and coming to accept physical and sexual limitation. Strikingly, the male-authored iron lung stories have more to say about disabled sexuality—both its successes and disappointments—than any narratives encountered in this research that were authored by polio-affected men who regained wheelchair or crutch mobility or made full recoveries. For multiple reasons, the iron lung narratives are the strongest—most moving, arresting, and transforming—in the polio nonfiction cannon.

In *Looking Up*, Needham recalls the break-up of her marriage with strength and even—in long retrospect—good humor. If we wish Mason had had the courage to cut herself loose from her husband's dead weight years before their final separation, Needham discerns almost immediately that her selfish husband needs removing from the picture and needs to be fought for custody of their three children. While divorce and especially custody battles often favor women, due to traditional perceptions of their helplessness to provide for themselves and their more essential attachment to children, in the case of utterly paralyzed, iron lung-using Needham, her court victories were surely landmarks in women's and disability rights. Needham, like Mason, came from a privileged background, which enabled adequate housing and round-the-clock home care during long intervals in Needham's life when the state had only the public institution to offer. Even so, the transition to polio living is significant; Needham's parents rearrange their retirement to defend and support her, and Needham describes on several occasions having to remove the kitchen door in her spacious home simply to get her iron lung to the sink for hair-washing.

Needham's politics—indeed this is the most politicized narrative in the survey—are a striking mix: when she is not battling the state for a disabled woman's right to raise her children, she is voting for Republicans in local and national elections. Her traditionalism asserts itself through the narrative's main thesis: that, like all women of this era, she is fulfilled primarily through successfully raising her children (in her case, in the conservative Catholic tradition). In the story's striking final chapter, Needham ponders the day her children will marry and leave home and makes a radical suggestion for the future: a "national custodial association" through which "the helpless" like herself would be permitted to room in with care-giving families who would earn, learn, and benefit from the presence of a "custodial" in their homes.[85] Throughout the narrative, Needham argues persuasively for home-based care instead of institutionalization; the plan she outlines here is recognizable as a nascent mandate for total self-sufficiency, as advocated by the independent living movement in recent decades. Thus, Needham's fervent desire to be a mother who stays "home" to raise her children (as opposed to losing them, and her life, to institutionalization) is as traditional as it is cutting-edge; her frequent, unemotional use of the term "helpless"—a word that retains its melodramatic shading despite her no-nonsense tone—partakes of this same ambivalence.

The politics of Kathryn Black's narrative are personal and familial, but no less complex for the inward turn they take. As the small child of a polio-affected, respirator-requiring mother, Black brings to light the psychic suffering glossed over in Chappell's cheery references to Bea Wright's three boys. In her unflinching dissection of her parents' failed relationship, she faces realities Mason seemed unable to confront in her life or her life-writing. Where Lidunska and especially Needham bravely, almost cheerfully, cut themselves off from their partners (in Lidunska's case, a fiancé, whom she freed from obligation by ceasing contact after polio onset), Black dwells movingly on the tragic loss of a father and provider who abandons his polio-affected wife and their children. As opposed to Charles Andrews's son Chuck, and Chappell/Wright's little Tommy, both of whom evidently fared well with physical and emotional separation from parents during a polio crisis, Black rails against the code of "no time for tears" that shielded children from sick parents (or sick children from parental comforting), the reality of pain and death, and hard truths. Her writing is an effort to recover the story that was denied to her when it happened, and the emotional scars she carries because of her traumatic separation from her mother motivate these moving accounts.

Black's mother Virginia contracted the virus when Black was only four years old and died two years later, death being an especially taboo topic within the canon of polio memoirs. As did Wright and Lidunska, Virginia suffered from the extremely dangerous bulbospinal form of polio, but Black's sense of its tragedy could not differ from Chappel/Wright's more strikingly: just for starters,

> As paralysis overtook Mother, aides lifted her onto the bed of an iron lung, on hand for just such an emergency. They carefully straightened her body and rolled the cotlike slab into its cylindrical tank, clamping it shut tightly. The rubber collar around her neck prevented air from es-

caping, and cotton padding reduced chaffing as the rubber slid up and down her neck with each breath. Her shoulders wedged against one end of her tank, her feet set firmly against a foot board at the other, she lay entombed, but alive.[86]

Later, "Mother hovered near death for days, her temperature and blood pressure dangerously high. She received around-the-clock care, but no medications could check the progress of poliovirus, and no doctor dared give a barely breathing patient a sedative or painkiller. All her attendants could do was suction her fluids, monitor her breathing, and wait for the crisis to pass."[87]

Following stabilization, Virginia seems to face a life of permanent total paralysis, the situation worsened by Black's emotionally and physically distant father, Dell. Clearly unequipped to handle his wife's catastrophic illness, he seeks out jobs in other states and stays out at night drinking when with the family. As Black sees it, "My father begged for a way out instead of insisting, willing Mother to live";[88] "he prayed each night, to a God he had no confidence in, for his death or Mother's."[89] Even as an adult, Black must deal with her father's insistence that her mother's was a "hopeless" case and wonder forever whether a different attitude would have led to a different outcome. Primarily, young Kathryn and her brother Kenny are raised by grandparents and live in an orphaned state, despite both parents' being alive. After many difficult months at home, with her aging grandparents struggling to care for her, Virginia dies, and Black's father leaves the family for good.

Even lovely Bea Wright was abandoned by a man at least once in her life; the father of her three children was evidently an unsavory figure whom Bea was right to divorce. Meanwhile, the remainder of her story stands apart from the other women-authored texts considered here for her striking good fortune (literally) in her dealings with the opposite sex. All of the others are eventually abandoned by husbands (and sometimes fathers) too weak to deal with their wives' (or daughter's) physical imperfections and limitations: Lidunska's narrative contains no mention of reattaching after letting her fiancé go; Mason is emotionally quitted upon by first father then husband; Needham, Black's mother, and Black herself are physically threatened and emotionally bereft when the husband/father takes flight. These abandoned women thus confirm Fairchild's thesis regarding disabled women's struggle for marital success, yet perhaps even more interesting is the striking range of responses to this situation, the opportunity the man's departure sometimes presented for the polio-affected woman to discover feminist inclinations and stretch protective wings around surviving loved ones including herself.

From the textual evidence, male iron lung survivors are luckier in love than their female counterparts; some who are single at polio onset find loving marital partners, often their nurses and therapists, despite quadriplegia and respirator requirement, while those who are married remain so, even if the sexual aspect of their partnership tragically never resumes. The many male-authored narratives of this subgenre are refreshingly willing to ponder post-impairment sexual desire—how strong it continues to be, despite the enervation of most other bodily movement and function. Sexual frustration takes on new meaning when the reader is forced to deal, alongside these authors, with the inability to even take the hand of a devoted spouse or charming nurse who has kindled the narrator's passion, much less relieve sexual tension with the consolations of masturbation, due to both lack of movement and lack of privacy in the hospital and also post-hospital settings. These authors convey the crushing disappointment of having a desirable loved one so near yet permanently unwilling to resume sexual contact. While they are vitally supported by spouses devoting themselves entirely to the improved personal and financial survival of the husband-narrator, the wives' inability to give or receive sexual satisfaction in the marriage indicates a tragic loss for both partners.

Resembling the collaborative partnership between Jim Marugg and Anne Buck Walters above, Mark O'Brien and Gillian Kendall co-wrote *How I Became a Human Being* (2003), O'Brien's story of his life as a polio-paralyzed quadriplegic. Kendall's role is in part explained by the fact that O'Brien passed away four years before the book was published, but not before the film made about his life, Jessica Yu's *Breathing Lessons: The Life and Work of Mark O'Brien*, won the 1996 Academy Award for Best Documentary (Short Subject). As in the case of Marugg and Walters, O'Brien's willingness to cowrite with a woman correlates with a refreshing focus on his physical and sexual self. Even pre-polio, in early childhood, O'Brien's overfed, overweight, frequently bullied and pummeled body is a recurring subject, as is his enjoyment of the sensual qualities of the water at the beach.[90] Post-infection/impairment, O'Brien comfortably relates his early masturbation experiences, despite the embarrassment these incidents originally induced. As a grown man, he hires a "sexual surrogate" with whom he has three sexual experiences and gains confidence; by the end of the narrative, he has found not only professional fulfillment as a journalist and poet but happy couplehood with Susan, although perhaps out of regard for her privacy, the only details about the relationship are conveyed in poetry each writes for the other.[91]

Louis and Dorothy Sternberg's *View from the Seesaw* (1986) is likewise remarkably frank, with respect to both the details of his sex life and, alas, the depths to which respirator-requiring Lou Sternberg has sunk to manipulate, exploit, and demean his self-sacrificing wife. It seems likely that Dottie resumed her role as Lou's sexual partner *only* because social custom dictated that she do so, yet certainly it is less Lou's physical condition than his controlling, abusive manner that must have been exceedingly difficult to set aside on the occasions of their sexual activity following his return from the hospital. One appreciates Sternberg's willingness to admit to the range of tactics used (and still in use) to keep his wife almost constantly on hand—feigning a crisis just as she was tending a child or going out, spoiling numerous family trips due to excessive fears of power outages in his breathing equipment, once even spitting in his wife's face. Yet one is simultaneously appalled at the misogynist ingratitude dealt out and endured in this remarkable, remarkably troubled marriage: "my children were so sweet, and I was so rottenly jealous and competitive and possessive of Dottie, who was trying to take care of all three of us. . . . At the point when I began to call her Mommy, David and Susie, who were seven and five, began to call her Dottie."[92]

Reminiscent of the gender dynamics that configured Charles Andrews's family, Lou comes from a patriarchal clan whose father and uncle visit the hospital frequently and prevent Lou's mother from doing so. She was "supposed to be too frail to bear the sight of me in the iron lung. She had always been overprotected and subservient to her husband"[93] and even after Lou's improvement and return home plays almost no role. Like many fathers on view in this survey, Lou's has great difficult dealing with his son's permanent impairment, changing into a "sad and bitter" man;[94] still Lou regards him as his "best friend" and comes to depend on the clout wielded by him and his uncle to get by in the hospital and do well in his business as a salesman-by-phone following release. Meanwhile, Dottie, who had been "rather quiet and shy" as a young married woman,[95] developed strength and assertiveness in the hospital and insisted on being Lou's primary, and often sole, caretaker once at home. Though Dottie no doubt enjoys her newfound roles of nurse, advocate, and business partner, they ultimately limit and exhaust her, as both she and her husband come to agree that only she knows how to properly care for him and thus must spend almost every minute of her life doing so.

While Lou is passionately preoccupied with his wife even while acutely ill—"along with all the infections, I had erections"[96]—he is also attracted to the nurses, whose intimate ministrations regularly turn him on and must be doused, literally, with pans of cold water to the groin. In one remarkable passage, Sternberg describes being so afraid of being turned by orderlies that he "crapped all over the place. I could feel it all over my legs and sheets. I smelled like a sewer."[97] This humiliating scene gives way almost immediately, however, to scenes of sexual arousal at the hands of his nurse Doris with whom he was "half in love" even though he longs for privacy with his wife who could then "relieve" him.[98] This striking mix of the scatological and sexual speaks both to Sternberg's overbearing, possessive attitudes toward his wife—note the same role played by the missing bedpan and the missed wife in these adjoining scenes—and to his great dexterity as both a writer and a polio survivor to take in, and write through, the most humiliating and "agonizing"[99] aspects of his situation in rapid yet honest fashion. Later he is embarrassed to have to use the bedpan in front of brusque, critical nurses;[100] at such moments we may recall the humiliations suffered by Hugh Gregory Gallagher and the connections made in his narrative between manual disimpaction in the hospital and sexual inhibition later in life. Luckily, Sternberg found himself for the most part in a much more supportive environment; his loss of bowel control impinges neither on his ability to enjoy sex with his wife—the only moments he forgets his pain and paralysis[101]—nor to tell a moving story of illness and recovery.

Resumed sexual activity is not part of the post-polio narrative, nor do the wives come off as heroically, in memoirs by Larry Alexander and Kenneth Kingery. Both accounts deal directly with what may be considered the death of their respective spouses' sexual desire when each man returns from the hospital emaciated, paralyzed from the neck down, and in need of a rocking bed. When Alexander confronts his wife with his physical desire for her, "she burst[s] out, jumping to her feet[,] 'It would be like sleeping with a corpse!'"[102] This is the last word on this subject, leaving the impression that the couple never resumes sexual contact. Kingery provides a similar scene[103] and a similar lack of resolution. In addition, it is Fran's parents who take control once Ken returns home, running the house and children without seeking his input. While still at the hospital, Ken labors to improve his respirator-free breathing time, which he builds up to eleven and twelve hours a day, despite the fact that these sessions include such straining of the chest and accessory neck muscles that passages describing them are painful to read. Kingery conveys the dynamic between himself and his disappointed wife perfectly, when she sweetly expresses her displeasure at his slow progress:

> "I don't understand," she said one day. "Way back before New Year's you were making fifteen-minute stretches. You're still only in the twenties."
> "I don't know, honey," I said, avoiding her eyes. "I'm—working a little all the time on the bed, you know."
> "So you should be getting stronger. Your time should be going *up!*"
> "The—bed doesn't have the same power as the iron lung," I blurted. "I'm afraid of—of getting overtired."
> She gazed at me for a long time, squeezing my hand. I had the distinct feeling I'd been a bad boy. Finally, her face tried to smile, but her words came cool. "Tired? When you're lying there resting most of the day and all night long? I don't like having to push you, Sweetheart. If you work hard enough yourself, you're bound to sleep at night."
> I thought to myself, "Or die of exhaustion."[104]

Later, Ken himself embraces unassisted breathing, taking big leaps in his endurance time whenever inspired by love from or for his family and friends. He even buys into a plan proposed by two high school friends—who "could only see me as Ken Kingery the athlete"[105]—to visit a miraculous doctor in the Chicago area, although it is this doctor who, admitting defeat, finally causes Ken to realize the permanence of his condition. Despite this psychological setback, Ken socializes with these friends and his wife without the respirator, feeling his most normal while chatting on the couch with them, sleeping over at their house, even having dental work done in an ordinary dental chair. Despite these and many such "victories" in the able-bodied sector, Kingery is never rewarded with the resumption of sexual activities with his wife. They share a platonic bed while visiting friends (and sleep separately while at home), never moving beyond the hand-holding stage.

Recurring feelings of alienation constitute the subtext of advocacy in the narrative. Kingery laments the outpouring of praise and sympathy for his saintly wife and instructively informs the reader that "No one told Fran how lucky she was to have such a masculine, good-looking, personable, cheerful, cooperative, hard-working, adoring husband."[106] These are all words that accurately describe the narrator in this story and all sentiments surely lost upon the able-bodied well-wishers who looked in upon and unfairly assessed this marriage. Later he critiques, through pity, the ableists who disable him: "These unfortunate souls spread a man's handicap all over him like butter on bread. They cluck their tongues and gush how nice that he can be at home with his loved ones. And they can't conceive how his mind—just lying there—can possibly come up with anything worthwhile."[107] Unfortunately, Fran herself is one of these disabling disbelievers for many pages into the narrative. Finally it is Kingery's son who takes time to locate and, following his father's instructions, install the microswitch that Kingery, trained in electronics through the military and in business, eventually uses to turn pages, answer the phone, and tape record letters to friends, feature articles, and his autobiography. As with Needham above, Kingery's conservatism fuels his recovery: his desire to instill traditional values in his children leads him to assert his role as authority in the family;[108] once his wife and in-laws are in his corner, his fears of juvenile delinquency and communist takeover at the hands of Nikita Khrushchev inspire his first articles, which lead eventually to his career as a freelance journalist.[109] Significantly, it is Kingery's right-oriented politics, and the cultural conservatism of many of the writers of these rocking bed narratives, that marks them as typical products of their era. Their normalcy makes its own statement even as it combines in remarkable ways with the radicalism occasioned by their disability.

Fiction and History

As worthy as is Kathryn Black's story for the events it recounts, perhaps it is even more significant to this discussion for all that is left out. Her struggle to "remember" her mother's young adulthood and especially her last two years opens onto the issue of fiction as it shapes and resurrects history in polio narratives. As a genre, memoir presents auto/biographical detail limited and redefined by faulty human brain chemistry (not to mention the memoirist's artistic license), yet great value inhered in postwar polio texts' *testimonial* status;[110] their authors had faced polio and lived to tell about it, their very writings serving as "proof positive" that one can tell an optimistic story about a terrifying disease.[111] More recently, new historicist critical methods have called into question authentic records of every kind, causing readers to consider the forces of indeterminacy and falsehood that underlie every gesture of historical representation. Especially those postwar narratives that sugarcoat what must have been a radical illness experience must be taken by contemporary readers with the proverbial grain of salt; the "proof" these midcentury texts offer is of the specific pressures brought to bear on the pop literature market of that period. Only inadvertently does "the truth" come out: male patients commenting on nurses' looks in their presence, frustrated doctors stamping out cigarettes on hospital floors. These remarkable social codes were surely enacted on a regular basis fifty years ago, and we are indebted to writing from this period for recording such incidental gems for posterity.

Above I considered various fictionalizations of the polio experience that serve neither writer nor reader especially well. Here, I am interested in specific instances of interpolated information into the historical record—the ways in which both Chappell and Black, for instance, insert non-biographical material to complete their stories—with markedly different results—and the ways in which Charles L. Mee, a playwright and a polio memoirist as talented as is Black, purposely interposes such material to enlarge the discursive effect but also, like Chappell, to shield his subject (in this case, himself) from full disclosure. Significantly, there is once again a sex-based component to these findings: the two women authors, Chappell and Black, so happen to be outsiders to the story they tell; that is, they are polio biographers, not autobiographers. Chappell may have had access to details that her narrative is simply in denial about, while Black was denied access to important parts of her mother's (and thus her own) story because of her young age and, I would argue, her female sex. Coincidentally, it is the male author, Charles Mee, who is in total command of the facts of his story but chooses to deny his reader access to some of these, especially those regarding what seem to be some turbulent years of his adult life.

Chappell employs the "new journalist" technique of making up the dialogue and incidental action of scenes from which she was absent. Because she is silent on the nature and extent of her source material, a safe assumption is that a heavy layer of fabrication has been thrown over a known narrative skeleton: even had Wright been able to recollect for her biographer a scene-by-scene reconstruction of the days before, during, and after her illness, surely she would have been unable to recall the long speeches and dialogues mouthed by the characters of her story, which Chappell has certainly simply filled in. From fabricating dialogue, it is only a short step to shaping and embellishing internal monologues, characters' emotional reactions to difficult situations. Thus, above, I referred to Chappell "forbidding" Bea to have a negative attitude about her mother's coldness; her true feelings are lost forever, and all we have is Chappell's heavy-handed rendition.[112]

By contrast Black and Mee deal powerfully with the significance of polio in their lives, blending history and fiction in similar ways to tell different stories and achieve different ends. While Mee, who cites Black and is influenced by her method, adds a stylized (i.e., fictionalized) strain of historical narrative to his own well-remembered story, Black deals dramatically with the need for polio writers to fictionalize certain aspects of a history whose loss is profoundly felt. While Mee calls on polio-related historical overviews and the polio memoirs of other survivors to supplement a life story whose thinness results from details (whole decades, in fact) that Mee prefers not to share, Black uses these same techniques to fill in a story she would love to share with her audience but cannot.[113]

Arnold Beisser questions the polio-affected person's over-reliance on memory, of a self it is impossible to recapture, as a form of denial.[114] Yet Mee complicates this sentiment by drawing simultaneously on history's two meanings: the past (i.e., his pre-polio physical state) and the actual (i.e., the reality of his polio-affected present). Adjusting to his home environment following release from the hospital, Mee benefits greatly from his role as a "historian," "someone who lived at least part in his memory, feeling it vividly, able to project myself back into a football game, a locker room, the feel of the padding, the sweat, the showers,"[115] but balances these reveries with reality-checking looks in the mirror[116] and a familiarity with the "facts" of his new body that he *also* defines as history: "At that moment, too, like a historian, I had become riveted by the facts of life. . . . From head to toe, from strong jaw to drop foot, I could see what I had to work with; I could count each robust and atrophied muscle.[117] History, then, is a concept including the (lost, pre-polio) past and the stark realities of the present (and future), the fiction of a former self that keeps one going (denial) and the reality of the mirror's image that balances our dreamlike tendencies (acceptance).

As affecting as is this image of the young boy caught simultaneously between past and present, competing versions of the historical, both of which will enable him to survive, the narrative's temporal leaps introduce an element of the ahistorical: moving slowly from the year of his infection (at age 14) to his graduation from high school, Mee watches himself cross the threshold of Harvard Yard, then moves the story into his successful present as New York playwright and instructor at Brown. Yet as the narrative draws to a close, the reader hears, in a single sentence, about Mee's "years of heavy drinking, some drugs, a fall into very deep depression, the love of more than one woman, three failed marriages, [and] a passionate life of writing history books that finally seemed pointless in their pretense."[118] When we learn that the drinking may be a direct reaction to the polio experience, stemming as it did from the "delinquency" Mee engaged in as soon as he regained enough physical mobility,[119] we sense that not only much of the life but even much of the polio experience is denied the reader in this narrative.

The most heart-rending aspect of Black's story—her extremely young age at the time of her mother's sickness and death—is that which most incapacitates her as she struggles to reconstruct the past. With the help of an older cousin and staff members and former patients from her mother's rehab center, Black pieces together her mother's story: her extreme physical situation, her deep depression, her failed marriage, and her post-polio failure to "be there" for her children to whatever degree she could. Many of Black's family members (e.g., her father and grandparents) are reluctant to dredge up these painful memories, and the reader shares the frustration of counting on these figures for vital details and meeting with resistance. Meanwhile, even helpful sources create the unpleasant sensation (for the reader if not for the author) of spoon-feeding Black her own past. As Black acknowledges about her cousin, "Katherine's stories offer me views of my mother and her life that otherwise would be lost to me. In her affectionate shaping of the anecdotes, I can also see myself as a child who had a mother and who was loved by her and by others. Once, when I asked, she wrote a letter giving me some memories."[120]

Such memories come even from accounts of other polio survivors, whose details Black overlays onto her mother's own story, so affecting are these accounts and so reliable are they in telling the *same* story, despite background differences. Black notes, "I couldn't separate those stories from my mother, and in reading each one, I unwillingly substituted Mother for each severe case."[121] Late in the text she even mentions putting an ad in the paper, as if shopping for "memories of polio."[122] Almost perversely, and in keeping with the efforts of the adults in her childhood to shield her from the worst, Black's own recollections are always in the wrong place at the wrong time: "I don't remember the newspaper reporter or photographer and have only a faded memory of Mother in the iron tank, but what I clearly recall about that Sunday in Denver was being outside the hospital, waiting."[123] Inexplicably, her memory improves as soon as her mother is gone: "but the time after her death, even the first years, are much more clear and whole in my mind. With Kenny on the top bunk and me on the bottom, we resumed our lives."[124] The spottiness of her recollection means that for pages at a time, Black's mother is "paralyzed" in some attitude of illness or rehabilitation, while Black fills in the gaps with responses to others' personal narrative and the public history of polio: the Sister Kenny, Roosevelt/Warm Springs, March of Dimes, and Salk vaccine stories. In cliff-hanger fashion, Black leaves her mother at death's door or tipping endlessly on her rocking bed for long recesses with these historical overviews that, while engagingly rehearsed, can only seem less urgent by comparison.

Black personalizes her contact with other polio auto/biographers, almost fictionalizing a relationship between total strangers and herself through her informal modes of referencing them. The author of *Flying Without Wings*, for example, seems to be someone she simply knows: "Arnold Beisser, a recent graduate of Stanford University Medical School and a national tennis champion when he got polio in 1960, was in an iron lung from the first moments of his illness."[125] The effect is augmented by the editorial decision to cite these sources only at the back, foregoing the superscript numbering system that would connect the reader to the relevant endnote, but that would also interrupt the intensely personalized (i.e., fictionalized) flow of the narrative.

Mee relies on many of the same stories to interrupt his personal narrative; perhaps because fiction and history are so inextricably bound for this author, he makes almost plagiaristic use of the sources he borrows from, purposely mislabeling print citations as anecdotes shared by visitors to his hospital room, personal friends, anonymous encounters in his life. Mee includes the account of "one boy" who is in fact Robert F. Hall, whose story I cite at the beginning of this book. He quotes freely from Edmund J. Sass's interviews and relates a story someone "told him" about a large bug dropping into the water-therapy tank of a paralyzed boy, which is actually a scene from page 70 of Wilfrid Sheed's polio novel, *People Will Always Be Kind*.[126] Like Black, Mee saves the intrusive textual references for the book's end, but is looser in his technique than even Black is; instead of the line-by-line references found in Black, Mee runs together the names of all his sources (excluding Sheed's, for some reason), in one large "Notes" section.

Thus, a polio memoir's fictional embellishments may take artistic license so far as to threaten the integrity of the memoir's testimonial properties (for instance in Chappell's case), or they may ultimately strengthen the narrative through creative, dramatic, immediate language. Black and Mee deploy artistic license with dramatic effect; Mee hides parts of his past (his personal history) behind other historical figures (especially other polio memoirists) transformed into fictional characters, while Black does not hide the fact that her own past is riven with blindspots and must be supplemented—and is powerfully supplemented—with what are both others' truths and a fictionalized biography of her own mother. In the same vein, the polio memoir's historical aspects may refer to the ancient history of the memoirist's pre-polio past, a zone of able-bodied reverie whose seductive draw, Beisser warns, can paralyze with denial. Meanwhile, again, especially for Black, the elusiveness of certain memories—those embedded within an intensely polio-affected past—become historical, remembered history, if and when they are successfully retrieved. Or the historical can simply refer to one's actuality, one's lived present, as is the case with Mee, who gazes objectively into the mirror and takes stock of his post-polio assets and liabilities. A simple equation of denial with either fiction or history is therefore impossible, though in general deploying fiction as history (as with Chappell) seems to take a text further in the direction of denial, while repackaging history as fiction (as with Mee and Black) constitutes the more radical method that enables the more creative, productive inquiry into the past.

Depression and Denial

At the outset, I considered the enigma of "denial," its mysterious transformation in a patient's course of recovery from rejuvenating positive outlook to disabling psychological "crutch." I questioned how a polio patient or therapist could ever know when denial had reached its maximum therapeutic potential and noted that for each person recovering from polio this maximum will be reached at a different point in the process. The issue is complicated when we recognize the phenomenon of "reverse denial" in play for some recovering from polio, for instance iron lung users, who may underestimate their ability to resume life outside the respirator. Some of its less common nicknames, "the iron cradle" and "the steel cocoon,"[127] indicate the emotionally complex response felt toward this apparatus by polio-affected respirator users, and the possibility that denial, working in concert with a preservation instinct already on high-alert, can leave the question of a patient's actual physical need for the iron lung unanswered. Also we have begun to discern, and will see in some of the texts discussed below, that denial is often less a problem for the polio-affected person than for friends and family members, as was the case, for instance, with Mary Grimley Mason and her father, who would not give up. This author and others in the genre indicate that denial in this form is readable as ableism itself. Analyzing cancer pathographies, Anne Hunsaker Hawkins identifies a "pathological syndrome" of denial, affecting every character in some of the texts she analyzes,[128] indicating that denial in its various manifestations is so contagious as to infect everyone associated with the illness/impairment experience.

Thus, in the mature stages of polio recovery, how does one differentiate (to oneself or to the rest of the world) the smiling face of denial from the smile of informed, serene acceptance, and how does one locate the point past which healthy grieving for one's physical losses becomes a paralyzing depression? As Wilfrid Sheed phrases the problem in the introduction to his polio memoir, *In Love with Daylight*, "The sugar-coating of pain is such an industry in America that you have to be twice as convincing as usual when you want to sell *real* sugar."[129] The authors to be considered here write in diverse and significant ways on the many directions one's emotional life might take, following survival of polio's acute infection and emergence into any combination of several permanent conditions. Significantly, each of the texts solicited for participation in this discussion, save one brief example (from Black), also happens to be male-authored; with one other exception (Milam's), each of the male-authored texts takes pains to theorize the phenomenon of denial itself, and each author-subject is a man who has enjoyed great professional (and sometimes personal) success yet whose relationship to denial, whose debt to denial, if you will, is one met with ambivalence. In short, each is, in Hugh Gregory Gallagher's terms, a "super-crip" whose memoir describes a career of impressive achievement but for whom subthemes of physical testing (even punishment), being "too hard one oneself" (both physically and emotionally), and the complex phenomenon of achievement itself all have special meaning. At the outset of the polio experience, denial is essential to survival. In their separate writings, Kathryn Black and Leonard Kriegel have attested to the healing powers of denial. Black laments her mother's failed "internal regulator," her inability to "deny her condition sufficiently,"[130] while Kriegel notes: "At the age of eleven, I needed to weather reality, not face it. And to this day, I silently thank those who were concerned enough about me, or indifferent enough to my fate, not to tell me what they knew."[131] Post-polio syndrome expert Lauro S. Halstead, M.D., describes the "mixed blessing" of denial (or "magical thinking") in the course of his own recovery from polio. He credits it for his "complete but miraculous" recovery[132] yet also faults it for the "negative lessons" many polio survivors are forced to learn: "We developed a strong denial system that has kept many of us distanced from the voices of our bodies. We are horrified and outraged at the possibility of being sick again [with post-polio syndrome], and we don't want to know that what we worked so hard to achieve might be lost."[133]

Gallagher contemplates this very transition, from adolescent illness and recovery, to crutch- and wheelchair-use in adulthood, to new attitudes assumed with middle age. He divides his memoir into episodes pertinent to this discussion — twenty years of productive, globe-traveling work enabled (and thus, says Gallagher, invalidated) by denial; a crash into depression during which he quit his job, closed his doors, and did not leave his bed for several weeks; and a third period best characterized as a working-toward instead of a final discernment of acceptance. After many months in therapy, Gallagher comes to regard his work life as a form of "masochism," a period of running from his disability during which "I appeared cheerful but was unhappy. The appearance fooled family and friends and confused me badly."[134] Gallagher avers that he found "no pleasure" in his years of professional accomplishment, an argument undermined to some degree by his later admission that his adventures on the job in Alaska and Africa were "wonderful things to do. Some of them were exciting, some were fun, all of them interesting. I would not have missed them for the world."[135] As he reads his punishing workload as a denial of his illness, so he denied what health he had by denying himself any social, sexual, or personal pleasure: "Most ghastly of all, I had placed myself beyond human concourse. I was unworthy, like a leper in exile."[136]

Even his arresting account of illness onslaught (see my discussion above) betrays an outlook shaped by depression: Gallagher recalls, with outrage, that he had not been allowed to pull his own plug while back in the hospital.[137] In the second and especially third movements, Gallagher beats himself up for having, ironically, beat himself up — for having punished himself both physically and psychologically with what he regards as the absurd burden of not only surviving but succeeding. So intent, therefore, is this author to avoid the false consciousness that he defines as denial, the false consciousness that he feels has been his entire consciousness since the night of his polio diagnosis, that suicide (or the living death of total social detachment) remains an attractive alternative.

Gallagher's wearing of his physical situation with reticence, reserve, and masochistic endurance could not differ more from that of his Warm

Springs roommate and life-long friend Lorenzo H. Milam, whose polio memoir is confrontational, almost sadistically graphic. It is the second narrative in this survey to refer to polio-related death (Kathryn Black's being the first): in brief but moving detail, he narrates a beloved sister's succumbing, then turns to his own turbulent polio story for the remainder of the text. Perhaps the ideal example of Arthur Frank's "chaos narrative," Milam's ranting style makes free use of exclamation points and all-caps to shout at his reader, and deploys repetition, attempting to convey yet more high emotion, ad infinitum: "She will get me up on my feet, up on my feet, standing on my own feet (not someone else's). It is Greta who will teach me, who will teach me, at last, after all this time, who will teach me."[138] Milam records explosive anger and agonizing pain with vivid immediacy and lingers over the polio patient's catheter-shredded urethra, bowel constipation, and oozing bedsores. While both Gallagher and Milam are frank regarding the details of their physical travails, Gallagher's anguished recollection contrasts with Milam's tone of near-enjoyment of subjecting the reader to the most jarring details of his recovery.

Where Gallagher withdraws from personal encounters, Milam pushes others out of his way. Post-rehabilitation, he reads all approaches to his situation as forms of denial; anyone who gets the door for him or helps him from a chair is making matters worse, and all verbal acknowledgments, from commendation for handling his crutches well to honest questioning by a relative's child, raise his ire. Milam basically accuses childhood friends of "remembering" him as an able-bodied boy (96) and rails against his mother for "weeping over" his transformed body,[139] rejecting heartfelt regret about his condition as vigorously as cheering denial. Only the mother of a friend from Warm Springs offers him solace: "She was one of my people, one of my new people, one of my post-inferno people. She isn't one of those people who will remember me running the stairs at age seventeen. She won't ever look at me with the I-remember look."[140] Can these figures from Milam's former life in fact be blamed for simply having known-him-when, and can Milam's desire to cut himself free of his past be read as a step toward acceptance and psychic healing? Certainly, the author's severe emotional reaction to family and old friends, and the author's own pointed refusal to deny his negative feelings, indicates that the answer to both questions is yes and no.

At his brother's wedding reception, he is accidentally knocked over by a new in-law and pulled to his feet by the apologetic crowd, entirely against his will. In this striking account, Milam wishes he could simply lie there, left alone, absenting himself from the vertical world of the able-bodied, who flow with ease all around him. His prostrate condition calls a realistic halt to his own charade of verticality, and could potentially cause all those around him to confront the profoundly disconcerting difference between themselves and this "horizontal man."[141] Such bracing realism, however, has its dark side, which Milam in a powerful reverie longs to embrace: "I am sorry that I thought, for a single moment, that I could leave the isolation and darkness of my bedroom, with its comfortable wheelchair and its long dark desk, and come all these uncomfortable miles so that I could go into my spectacular collapsing act with perhaps thousands of guests. I am sorry to have left my room and my desk, before which I could sit and stare at my hands, at my long, pale, white hands, where I could sit in the safety and security of my dark room and stare at my hands."[142] When his new family yanks him back "to life," to cover their own embarrassment more than anything else, they deny him the respite of a depressive lapse, in a manner likely to be applauded by psychotherapists, but completely disempowering to this patient in the process. Almost in reaction to this turning-point incident, Milam absents himself from his family, past, and home nation, spending the rest of his text among "new people" on a "post-inferno" plane of existence. Significantly, then, denial emerges in this text as acknowledgment, as all Milam's well-wishers fail in their very gesture of well-wishing, no matter how optimistically or pessimistically they do so. Milam refers to no social interaction during which his situation is actually ignored, leaving open the possibility that this approach, for this polio survivor at any rate, is preferred.

In the rejuvenating environs of Europe, Milam feels freer to not only be his disabled self but to explore his homosexuality, eventually selecting the most strapping young man from a parade of candidates culled from the impoverished local Spanish population to care for his "physical needs." The support he is seeking, however, pertains not at all to his physical disability—in fact Milam is largely self-sufficient—but to his long-contained desire to express himself sexually with another man. Thus Milam's reveling in social and sexual contact constitutes another point of opposition to Gallagher's career of ascetic self-denial,[143] yet Milam's admiration for the perfect physical form, as well as the ethnic and class privileges that enable him to travel as an exploitative sexual tourist among Spain's impoverished lower classes, manifests its own form of denial: has Milam not "learned" anything from his experience as a disfigured, impaired polio-affected person, with respect to applying elitist physical standards to prospective sexual partners, or is Milam unbounded by the mandate to learn anything from his impairment at all? Shall his rejection of several older and less attractive men who proposition him throughout Europe be regarded as an irony he fails to heed (i.e., a gesture of supreme hypocrisy) or is his rejection of unattractive able-bodied men in fact entirely different from an able-bodied man's rejection of him? Milam refers at one point to "my thin and bony leg,"[144] indicating that one leg is appreciably smaller than the other; the book's cover features a photograph of a man's legs, the left one of which is trussed up in heavy bracings. Yet the discomfort provided by the image of the apparatus is mitigated by the healthy, attractive legs of the model wearing it, whose brace is applied gratuitously—almost erotically, S&M style—and thus questionably.

As does Milam, Kriegel recognizes the value of anger in the spectrum of the polio survivor's emotional response, demonstrated by Milam throughout his raucous narrative and by Kriegel in his essay "A Few Kind Words for Anger." In it, Kriegel notes that, "When it is visibly displayed, anger makes us uncomfortable, for it reveals the self on the verge of moving out of control. Most Americans prefer to deny the existence of that self, or at least prefer to ignore it."[145] Kriegel's pointed word choice suggests that anger is a perfect analogy for impairment itself, public enactment of which is inappropriate (because unnecessary) for the able-bodied but perhaps for the paralyzed polio-affected person—since anger is a form of "movement"—the ideal liberating gesture. If, as Gallagher's story above implies, denial is a form of "running from" the problem of paralysis or other physical debilitation, anger may be seen to "move" a paralyzed body in a more favorable direction—up the scale of socially valuable entities, if it can move others to see it in fairer, more accepting ways.

Yet Kriegel's anger, credited with leading him directly from denial to "honesty," "acceptance," and "peace," must be read as at least in part its own form of denial. He determines at the moment of his anger-epiphany that "to be a cripple meant that the need to be a man was stronger and even more decisive"[146] than it was for ordinary men, and that "the determination to get even with 'my virus' was not as crazy as it sounded."[147] The desire to compete with able-bodied men and the antiviral revenge fantasies indicate that Kriegel remains far from accepting limitation, a measure of powerlessness in certain situations.

Charles L. Mee and Arnold Beisser examine yet another form of denial—a figurative severing of the body from the mind (or, literally, head) in the situation of polio-induced quadriplegia. Both Mee, who eventually regained upper body mobility, and Beisser, who remained paralyzed below the neck, contemplate a future lived entirely in the head, denying the presence, the meaning, the very life of the body—Beisser refers effectively to his as "it"—since it has indeed been transformed, more or less overnight, into an inanimate object. Mee's initial inability to lift his head, to even look upon his newly immobilized self, and Beisser's permanent loss of his own corpse-like corpus inside the coffin-like iron lung surely encouraged these writers further in their psychic deployment of this dichotomy. At its worst, Beisser's mind/body severance induced feelings of powerlessness: "Those who attended my body did things when and how they believed they should be done, and I seemed to have little or no part in this, except to feel the effect of what they did. They were not unkind, but they were more the owners of what lay inside the tank than I."[148]

Mee had been planning a football career, at least through college, and realized that "whatever vague plans I may once have had to make my way in the world with my body were now useless. Henceforth, I would have to use my head. And my head was empty. And so I filled it with Plato."[149] Elsewhere, "in the summer of '53, my mind simply left my body, and it never came back for good. My sense of who I am would never again reside in a body that let me down; it moved instead into a mind that promised to be more trustworthy, more devious and elusive."[150] Finally, "I don't have multiple personalities, but I do know that the body I move around and put here and there in the world is something separate from my self."[151] The "self" that has been cut off from the now failed body indeed has found, at least in the case of gifted writers like Mee, a productive, almost independent life of its own. Mee's reference to "multiple personalities," meanwhile, indicates the "schizoid" sensation surely experienced when separated so irrevocably from one's physical self—a disintegration radically liberating (from the philosophical perspective), yet threatening to one's mental "wholeness" as well.[152]

Beisser, who was both a finishing medical student and semi-professional tennis player when polio struck him as young man, is nothing if not philosophical about his marked physical impairment in the long view provided in *Flying Without Wings* (1989): the complicated thoughts he has arrived at within (and in many ways enabled by) his paralyzed state—literally, a philosophy of total paralysis—have produced a style of mind expansion that has allowed him to look with acceptance, even affection and love,[153] upon his impairment—"being philosophical" in a figurative sense. While he experienced, in the early years of impairment, a depressing, immobilizing narrowing of his world, Beisser describes the manner by which he entered into this limitation, enabling him to leave his physical situation behind. Where Sternberg referred to sex as the escape mechanism that enabled him to set aside his impairment, for Beisser, it is intense mental concentration or exuberant laughter—especially when shared with a colleague or his beloved wife—that "nurtures [me] back to health for the moment."[154] Elsewhere, "when I join with some other person or task and am fully absorbed, it is as though I have left my body and am but a pinpoint of awareness—aware only of this moment and this 'thing'. . . . Time and space are fused and my body seems to disappear. Time accelerates, so that I am identified with it, and I am time."[155] The "multiple personality" reference in Mee's text is re-envisioned here as a radical separation of the physical and spiritual planes that constitutes total enlightenment.

Thus we note the turn toward philosophy—the original life of the mind—in the comments of both these authors.[156] Mee relied on Plato, Aquinas, and classical history to excite his mental faculties, best peers and teachers when he returned to school, and inspire the plays he wrote later in life, many based on ancient Greek models. The themes in Beisser's narrative include time, space, and time-space relationships; he indicates that the fully immobilized are singularly resigned, and also singularly qualified, to ponder at length, and with terrific analytic payoff, life's basic mysteries.

In both cases, these writers' denial of their physical bodies recalls the frustrating failures to connect physically with others so helpfully broached by Gallagher above. If polio-affected quadriplegics like Beisser feel bound to vacate the body and move permanently into "the attic," as it were, even those with partially restored function such as Mee and Gallagher may renounce, by strict ascetic denial, sexual pleasure and even basic human contact. Shortly after discovering Plato, Mee recalls appreciating this philosopher for "the dialogue form, the opposing arguments, the turmoil of conflicting ideas and feelings; he spoke to my own warring mind and heart."[157] Mere hours after taking leave of the body that has in fact abandoned him, Mee recalls for the reader—if not for himself at that moment—that despite the immobilized limbs, trunk, and spine, the "heart"—the vital organs, the need for love, the bodily appetites and lusts—beats on. Thus, bodily denial such as the kind Gallagher described may be seen as doubly formed—denial that the incapacitated parts had stopped working, denial that the still-working parts (especially "the heart") yet required his attention. Both Mee and Beisser seem to have had more success in such matters of the heart: Mee married three times and, according to his autobiography, currently enjoys a loving relationship, while Beisser and his physical therapist fell in love shortly into his convalescent phase and remain happily married at the end of his memoir.

While Milam and Kriegel describe "anger" as an effective vehicle to an emotional state of acceptance of their disability, Mee regards it as a "waste of valuable energy,"[158] and Beisser, as indicated above, instead credits humor with curative powers. His upbeat perspective even includes striking personifications of his impairment, as he gives it the body it has taken from him. At one point it is a "Roshi, a little Zen master, who is always with me, enigmatically smiling at my struggles."[159] Elsewhere,

> Frequently, I see my disability . . . as an adversary, an opponent or an enemy to be overcome and battled with. This is very useful for me sometimes, and allows me to try to compete against it, to try to beat it, and gives me a clear focus for my effort. It is interesting that when I think of my disability as an enemy, it is a male adversary. I try to face him squarely to look at him in the eye, and to hold my ground. . . . When I accept my fear, I accept and respect the power of my opponent, and he no longer dominates me. We join together. When I do surrender, my disability becomes female, and we are united in that special way that men and women can unite. We are in confluence, and the relationship is perfect. We are in agreement.[160]

Note the nuanced sense of taking on his disability that contrasts with Kriegel's somewhat overconfident stance above. The battle is joined only "sometimes," under certain circumstances, and Beisser's many references to "trying" indicates his clear awareness that this will be no easy victory. In fact, there will be failure on many occasions, and Beisser's imaging of the conquering disability transforming into a heterosexualized female "partner," whom he does not feel humiliated by but instead embraces, is its own form of victory. Acceptance of disability seems less locatable in efforts to distract and ignore than in getting inside the impairment, as Beisser has done, understanding it as fully as possible (as only the impaired themselves can), and integrating it into one's daily routine, ordinary thought processes, and prospects for happiness and fulfillment. Beisser's personification of his impairment is a fitting example of Frank's ideal quest narrative: "Quest stories meet suffering head on; they accept illness and seek to *use* it. Illness is the occasion of a journey that becomes a quest."[161]

Conclusion

Echoing the sentiments of Arnold Beisser, Louis Sternberg notes that despite years of growing acceptance and many accomplishments (including success as a salesman in the garment business and a doctorate in linguistics from Brandeis), he "ha[s] some setbacks still, of course."[162] "I still cry now sometimes, for the same reasons, and there is an empty sinking feeling in the pit of my stomach if I let myself contemplate that this is going to go on for the rest of my life."[163] The "seesaw" of his memoir's title refers, thus, not only to the rocking bed that has assisted his breathing for the greater part of his life but also to the back-and-forth quality of his outlook from one day to the next, dependent upon numerous personal, familial, and social factors. Indeed many of these narratives indicate that adjustment to one's post-polio condition is not a state of serenity only achieved once crossed into confidently and permanently but an often provisional, temporary, and shifting outlook that is attained more easily and for greater periods with adequate passage of time and an adequate sense of personal fulfillment and/or social support. At the outset, I indicated how writing one's polio story militates against total surrender to depression, yet the polio survivor's testimonial is otherwise profoundly implicated as a gesture of both denial and acceptance. We have seen that many women and men authoring such texts have used the occasion of writing to maneuver around painful issues of disability, loneliness, disrupted gender roles, sexual unattractiveness, financial ruin, and abandonment by parents, spouses, or friends. Some have underestimated the level and complexity of their physical limitation—at least insofar as they decline to share a full exploration of same with their readers—while a few appear to have overestimated their disability through melodramatic stylistics or false-sounding recollections of their experience.

Midway in this chapter, I paired two woman-authored biographical accounts with starkly opposite outcomes—total vigorous restoration for the protagonist of Eleanor Chappell's memoir, agonizing loss and death for the protagonist of Kathryn Black's—and considered the markedly divergent ways in which each mingled "fiction" and "history" to create their testimonial accounts. In addition, these two texts cover the spectrum from the most tonally restrained to the most direct attempt to render the suffering endured by those surviving the loss of a loved one to polio. Chappell's privatization of Wright's experience—a tactic depicting polio contraction as so shameful an occurrence as to require almost complete avoidance of its details—confirms the concerns of disability theorists who reject the personal tragedy/heroic victory dichotomy perpetuated in such a story; meanwhile, Black's inclusion of multiple, collective, and personal polio "histories" effectively socializes the personal impairment experience, yet artfully recaptures the sense of individual and familial suffering, sadness, and loss that fully rewards our literary sensibility and suggests how remarkably eye-opening such individualized accounts can be. It is writing such as Black's that I have characterized as the "strong" response to polio, as Frank's "good story," regardless of whether authored by or on behalf of a woman or a man.

Once more, even the "weakest" among these works are valuable as conduits to the past and as testament to the extreme difficulty faced by any polio survivor seeking healthy self-acceptance in the life that must be lived and even in the story that must be told. The very nature of the polio memoir, its finite singularity as an individual work, dictates an ending (most often either sugar-coated or truly sweetened) that cannot help but misrepresent the ongoingness of polio-related impairment for an able-bodied readership; yet the most effective of these *do* manage to subvert the genre's formal mandate to close the book on the polio experience by crafting images and insights that permanently linger with and thus productively transform the previously uninitiated reader. Throughout this chapter, narratives by those most severely affected by polio's permanent effects were read as the strongest on the subjects of the polio experience, sex and disability, sexism and disability, the rights of the severely impaired, and the roles played by acceptance and denial.

When Carol Thomas argues that "the time has certainly come for disabled women to tell their stories,"[164] she indicates that such speaking out will end the silencing enforced not only by the able-bodied mainstream but also by indifferent feminist "sisters" who have ignored their disabled membership for too long and by (mostly male) "social-modellists" who insist that neither the individual account nor the physical body has a place in disability studies. While I have argued throughout this discussion that both men and women serve themselves and their readers best by telling their stories in no uncertain terms, Thomas's feminist take helpfully politicizes the problem: with respect to the polio memoir, there is less a divide between women and men than an ever-oscillating tension between stereotypically masculine and feminine approaches to the writing challenge. Those narratives that resist the upswinging tendency of "the comic plot" and play instead with daring variations such as persistent decline, jagged peaks and valleys, or frustrating stasis break loose of the structural patterns pervasive in the genre and avoid the pitfalls of denial as they do. As the strong, "manly" narrative of polio is its own Achilles heel, so the "weakness" evinced in other accounts is the genre's greatest strength.

3

"Crippled by History": Polio and the Past in Contemporary Novels

IN JAMES BALDWIN'S CLASSIC "SONNY'S BLUES," THE NARRATOR'S young daughter Isabelle contracts polio and dies in the story's prehistory. Central to the argument I will present in this essay is the situating of polio, in this story as in dozens of others, in the narrative *past*, yet also the way in which polio affects the narrative present in significant ways:[1] Isabelle's death causes the narrator to reunite with his estranged younger brother, Sonny, after many years, and references to the girl's death function structurally to move the story in and out of its excursions into the recent and distant past. As little Isabelle's polio is tragically signaled when she takes a serious fall, so Sonny is imaged as "falling" multiple times, linking him with the little girl and presenting the narrator with the profound challenge of catching him in time, as he was not able to do for his daughter.[2]

Unforgettable in many ways, Baldwin's story is significant here for being a work of fiction, a canonical work at that, dealing with polio *during* America's polio period: the middle decades of the twentieth century when infection rates were highest, the March of Dimes was little less than a national pastime, and the Salk vaccine was perfected (in 1955). Yet despite the structurally and thematically essential role played by polio in "Sonny's Blues," informal polling of colleagues and students indicates to me that it is a universally forgotten aspect of the story. Marc Shell has examined "the general repression of the memory of polio,[3] in contemporary America, observing that "the history of polio is the history of forgetting polio."[4] While polio was finally a fairly rare occurrence even during the peak years of the late '40s and early '50s, it remained an intractable medical mystery and a source of universal anxiety throughout this period. Yet as Shell observes, the polio experience was moved past almost as soon as it occurred: parents refused to share facts with their affected children; rehabilitation methods included "repression," "distraction," and "compensation";[5] and the immediate leave-taking of the illness itself with the advent of the Salk vaccine has caused, Shell argues, levels of ignorance and denial in the medical community that not only harm those now dealing with post-polio syndrome but very likely others with degenerative diseases (especially ALS), who might benefit from the discoveries continued study of polio might have afforded.

Shell's survey of polio fiction and memoir worldwide creates a particular picture; my focus on a specifically American literary canon (or "polio school")[6] indicates that postwar-era nonfiction accounts of the polio experience appeared in number enough to help launch the genre of the illness narrative, yet almost no fictional works were published before Wilfrid Sheed's *People Will Always Be Kind*, twenty years following the Salk vaccine—a cultural lapse that defies explanation.[7] Especially when we consider the wealth of novels and short fiction from this period treating in detail another national nightmare, the atom bomb, the lack of a literary response to polio is even more striking. Perhaps the boom in polio memoirs, as well as the complex narrative played out through awareness campaigns, fundraising appeals, and celebrity sponsorship promoted by the March of Dimes, mitigated the need for treatment of the subject in novels or films (where it was also rarely dealt with).[8] Even more importantly, the essential differences between fears of the bomb and of polio may offer a clue: atomic conflagration remained, for those in the West at any rate, a frightening but ultimately unrealized scenario that, had it materialized, would have stricken the nation collectively and completely. In terms pertinent to this discussion, the atomic threat remained in America's future, where it appealed as a subject to the authors of futuristic genres like science fiction and fantasy, as well as to progressives and other forward-thinkers who used their politicized fiction to help avert disaster. By contrast, polio belonged to the postwar present, striking individuals and families (instead of the entire nation in one blast) with such devastation that the fantastic genres (and even mainstream fiction) may have seemed frivolous and useless alternatives to the instructive, realistic narratives provided by popular journalism, polio-survivor memoirs, and March of Dimes information campaigns.

Indeed, the novelistic silence characterizing polio's own present (the immediate postwar period) has given way to a boom in fiction related to polio as *past*, that is, as an index of America's own "childhood," its seemingly simpler, more innocent era. As we might distinguish a quaint, bygone "atomic" moment from a nuclear threat still very much with us, so polio no longer belongs to the list of things from which Americans might take sick and die, and thus occupies a perverse position on the "life" side of the balance sheet—as a medical triumph, a false fear, an evocative literary device. While polio fictions of the historical-romance variety exploit an almost charming rendition of polio as temporalizing shorthand for the golden middle decades of the twentieth century,[9] others explore a distinctive configuration of the American historical—private or familial "ancient history," which lingers through the present like a permanent impairment; a specific decade from the national past; or identifiable historical markers (inter/national figures or incidents) that may either effectively counterbalance or thematically disrupt an elemental, "timeless" natural environment. From the academic snobs in Wallace Stegner's *Crossing to Safety*, utterly indifferent to the Nazi threat,[10] to the polio-affected characters in Michael Chabon's *The Amazing Adventures of Kavalier and Clay*, ready to give their lives to the defeat of Hitler, the blend of history with fiction in polio novels runs the gamut. And where the course of illness—onset, nadir, recuperation, rehabilitation—structures almost all polio memoirs, most of the novels considered here historicize polio by setting the illness itself firmly in the narrative past, focusing instead on the post-polio impairment experience in the private and social spheres.[11] As history, polio figures in these novels as both the past and the literal and entwines in interesting ways with its putative opposite, "the fictional"—which I will identify as both historically inaccurate (downplayed *or* exaggerated) portrayals of the polio experience and, more simply but quite differently, a well structured plotline.

Especially the issue of pacing—*movement*—in stories including characters hobbled by polio will be pertinent to this discussion, will require me to evaluate not so much the overall quality of the work in question (as in the typical book review) as the progress of the fictional narrative as this is enabled, obstructed, or obliterated by the presence of "history" (polio and other weighty subject matter) in these novels. Disability theorists David T. Mitchell and Sharon L. Snyder argue that physical difference is in many ways fundamental to narrative's progress: "it is the narrative of disability's very unknowability that consolidates the need to tell a story about it. . . . The effort to narrate disability's myriad deviations is an attempt to bring the body's unruliness under control."[12] Yet as correct as this may be in many cases, it is equally valid to question narrative for the countless occasions upon which it abandons its effort to know (or even control) disability by simply leaving it behind. Often disability is less an essential or obsessive theme than a device deployed variously throughout a narrative—at the beginning, "to provide highly visual *hooks*, to engage the audience's interest,"[13] at dramatic turning points mid-story, on intermittent occasions signaled by the arrival of a disabled minor character, or saved for a startling conclusion.[14]

Martin Norden describes the tendency of film to "isolate disabled characters from their able-bodied peers as well as from each other," using "framing, editing, sound, lighting, set-design elements (e.g., fences, windows, staircase banisters) to suggest a physical or symbolic separation of disabled characters from the rest of society."[15] Rosemarie Garland Thomson observes that "disabled literary characters usually remain on the margins of fiction as uncomplicated figures or exotic aliens," that "main characters almost never have physical disabilities";[16] finally, Lennard J. Davis argues that the genre of the novel itself, "that proliferator of ideology,"[17] "promotes and symbolically reproduces normative structures."[18] Many have equated illness with realism, while disability is gothic,[19] the grotesque,[20] and the uncanny.[21] Howard Brody deems literary examples "using sickness in a solely metaphoric manner" less relevant to his investigation,[22] but disability theorists[23] complain that metaphoric (poetic, inaccurate) treatments of disability are the *only* ones available in most literature. Mitchell himself, elsewhere reading the children's classic, *The Steadfast Tin Soldier*, observes that "once the soldier's incomplete leg is identified, the difference is quickly nullified.... In fact,...the figure undergoes a series of epic encounters without further reference to his limitation."[24] Mitchell points here to the catch-22 I discern hindering various contemporary novels including polio-affected characters: either the character must leave behind (i.e., relegate to his/her personal past) the disability in order to stay actively involved in the narrative or risk being left behind by the narrative itself.

Interestingly, Mitchell reads the tin soldier's adventures as Odysseus-like—heroic, harrowing, and a measure of his physical prowess—but in fact each is a passive assault upon his inert, impaired body (an observation admittedly complicated by the fact that this "body" is made of inanimate tin): "he falls out of a window, his bayonet gets stuck in a crack; a storm rages over him later that night; two boys find the figure, place him into a newspaper boat . . . he is accosted by a street rat."[25] In a troubling way, these several passively received (mis)adventures adhere faithfully to the limitations in question; they maintain the impaired soldier in a central role but deny him agency in every instance. In its ideal form, then, the polio novel would consistently engage its theme by enabling its polio-affected character(s) to carry a meaningful yet realistic share of the narrative itself. As historical fiction it would combine an invented narrative with a sweeping historical account: we recall that in addition to history meaning "the past" and "the literal," a third definition regards time itself: history discerned as the passage of time connotes its own form of movement, while dramatic or epic moments in history are indistinguishable from fiction's own "good story" (see chapter 2).

In fact, this ideal model remains largely that; in most polio novels the relationship is less than harmonious between the storyline and its various historical features: not only polio, rendered most often as an individual or familial issue, but also more collectively experienced phenomena such as the Roosevelt administration, race relations in the South, World War II, or the postwar partitioning of Berlin. In some polio novels, the ponderousness of historical information causes the core narrative to stumble to a halt; when a novelist succeeds in boring a reader thus, s/he indeed threatens to consign polio (and the other historical narratives cited) to the dustbin of history. Yet just as threatening to the history of polio—and to the physically impaired of the present day—is the narrative so caught up in the sweep of history-writ-large that the polio-impaired character is relegated to "minor" status or killed off by some handy device, allowing the narrative's able-bodied figures their unhindered dash toward the story's conclusion.

In Baldwin's story, the Isabelle subplot resonates thematically with the story's larger preoccupation with children and youth: the narrator teaches "boys" algebra in a public school, refers to Sonny's adult peers as "boys," and sees the lost child in the faces of his declining Harlem neighbors. The story ruminates on multiple mortal threats to the young in an impoverished urban context, including street violence, heroin, despair, and the early loss of one or both parents. Likewise, the polio canon in general plays upon the theme of childhood innocence, often keeping its juvenile characters "out of trouble" (i.e., out of the crises and epiphanies of childhood itself) or keeping its adult characters in a state of permanent childhood—disqualified for work, war, sex, or love. Disability theorists have documented the limitations placed upon the disabled (perhaps especially disabled women) with respect to free and full access to meaningful work, interesting leisure, and worthwhile marital and sexual prospects.[26] The infantilizing endured by polio characters is a form of isolation that contemporary readers may also (wish to) read as a relic of the past—a situation that modern medicine and technology, cultural attitudes, and educational opportunities are supposed to rescue the modern-day physically impaired from having to endure. To the degree that disabled Americans still face such isolation, arrested development, and enforced innocence, these more complex, less nostalgic treatments of the age of innocence contain a message of continuing relevance.

Meanwhile, accounts analyzed by Daniel J. Wilson in his recent *Living with Polio* indicate that in fact many polio survivors have enjoyed lives complete with rewarding careers, happy marriages, and sexual fulfillment;[27] reading their stories once again underscores the dichotomy between nonfiction and novels (the historical and the [mis]representative) that is an overriding theme in this chapter. Even polio novels that effectively critique polio-related infantilization may finally reinscribe the "minor" status of their impaired characters and must be questioned for this. Disability theorists' complaint against the relegation of the polio-impaired and other impaired to the status of "minor" character in some novels resonates here. Likewise, their arguments employing spatial concepts of marginality and othering have their temporal corollary in the persistent device of infantilization on display in several of the novels to be discussed: narratives that leave their polio characters behind may be said to outgrow these characters in unacceptable ways; in many novels to be considered below, the inherent boyishness of male polio-protagonists is emphasized, while female ones are killed off before the question of their sexual identity becomes a narrative stumbling block.[28]

The issue of homosexuality also occurs regularly in polio novels, a coupling perhaps not surprising when we consider their complementarity in this particular American context. In the middle twentieth century, homosexuality was a shameful, limiting "sickness" just as polio was, one we have also "recovered from" at last—though by vaccinating not against the "disease" but against our own perceptions of it as a sickness in the first place. While gay and lesbian literary figures are more and more ubiquitous narrative elements, "the homosexual," like "the atom bomb" and "the polio," is narrative shorthand by which an author can set his story in a particular past—the pre-1960 "age of ignorance" when—we now realize—homosexuality was the least of our worries. More directly, various of the novels discussed below show how polio can "queer" those it affects by removing them from the heterosexual marriage game, how polio, like homosexuality, pathologizes and infantilizes those it affects in terms of arrested sexual development, of permanent adolescence.

Thus in Jaames Carroll's *Secret Father*, Michael's weak, deformed legs not only make him self-conscious in front of girls like Kit; they also lead to his father's overprotective attitude and his suggestion that Michael major in "fine arts in college. You have the sensitivity for it." Michael "would choke on the words [he] was unable to utter: *Sensitivity. Since when is that something to put on your resumé? Since when is that a virtue?* Virtue, [he] would think then, from the Latin, meaning manly."[29] In both Dorothy Uhnak's *The Ryer Avenue Story* and Rona Jaffe's *The Road Taken*, the polio-affected protagonists grow up to be not wives but doctors, suspiciously mannish pursuits in the 1950s; Uhnak's Megan is even accused of lesbianism by her nemesis, due to her devoted attachment to Patsy, another tomboy, in her childhood. In the novels including the issue of homosexuality, I will continue to examine its relationship to polio below.

While the polio-affected characters in the dozens of novels I have researched on this subject in fact play major, active, sympathetic roles, the findings of disability theorists are borne out with respect to most of these stories' climactic moments and resolutions; many of these novels ultimately marginalize their polio characters, despite initial efforts to make them (and often their conditions) central to the action. This troubling pattern can only detract from these texts' otherwise valuable attempts to position polio—its cultural and conceptual significance—within the larger narrative of the American twentieth century.

Two Nonfiction Novels

Perhaps not surprisingly, many of the polio novelists discussed in this chapter experienced polio in their personal pasts, via their own infection or that of a loved one. Many, therefore, have written both fiction and nonfiction accounts of the polio experience or blend personal and public history, self-exposure and self-fashioning, in "nonfiction novels" (Sheed's term) that productively dimensionalize this canon. Sheed's *People Will Always Be Kind*, appearing as it did in 1973, literally functions as a bridge text between the run of polio memoirs appearing in the postwar period and the boom in polio-themed novels of 1990s to the present. Likewise the story itself transitions from a pseudo-memoir, which narrates the polio illness and recovery of young Brian Casey in moving detail, to a present-day account of the adult Brian as U.S. senator running for president but losing for enigmatic reasons. The question, as it will be throughout this chapter, regards the successful integration of this protagonist's past and present: does the novel's post-polio portion (and its adult protagonist) build upon its polio portion (and adolescent protagonist), or is there a general falling away from the theme and import of polio as the novel turns to other things? To begin to answer, my reference to the "moving detail" of the polio portion should be read literally: ironically, the narrative of Brian's halted personal development is dramatically enacted, psychologically complex, geographically wide-ranging, and buoyed along at every moment by bracing dark comedy.[30] This early story involves Brian's dogged search for full recovery; though the search fails, this hardly stops Brian, with legs in braces, from scholastic achievement and the realization in his early days among indolent, pretentious leftists at Columbia, that "left to themselves, [his friends] probably moved even slower than he did."[31] Yet here the story itself begins grinding to a halt; facing permanent disability, Brian discovers that he excels at speech-making, and the career of this gabby politician is born.

In the hands of speech-writer Sam Perkins (the narrator of the second half), Brian is no longer in sharp focus, and the effects of his earlier illness on the kind of man and leader he becomes are never clear. Instead, the narrative hunkers down to the minutia of backroom deal-making, debates, primaries, and conventions ad nauseam—again, losing the focus on Brian's character (especially as polio-affected) and lapsing from action to talk. Tension-building discoveries falter: Sam "certainly didn't expect" Brian's wife to say "My husband is a very great man"[32] at the end of their first interview, but what else is a politician's wife supposed to say? Later, he "gapes" when she reveals that her husband was lonely and shy when she met him,[33] but of course Brian's plainly visible impairment makes such a statement entirely plausible. Finally, Sam is shocked to learn that Brian tells lies,[34] yet lying is so endemic to politics that we again cannot see the basis for Sam's surprise, nor can we ascribe this vice to this particular politician's polio past. If in fact Brian determines to exploit his disability to win women, friends, and power (though no language in the novel indicates that it ever occurs to him to do so), why does Brian choke at story's end and lose the national election? Certainly, the political campaign is an intriguing terrain for a polio-affected character—you've got to have "the nerve"[35] and "the legs" to "run" for office;[36] yet the novel's sharp severance of past from present, both thematically and stylistically, means that Brian's ultimate loss (almost surrender) of the election may—or may not in the least—replicate and result from his earlier losses.

3 / "CRIPPLED BY HISTORY"   105

Polio memoirist-activist Anne Finger's *Bone Truth* (1994) tells the story of a pregnant, polio-impaired woman dealing with multiple personal crises and also declines to integrate polio into its own broader historical concerns (America's communist era) and its main character's self-realization. Ruminating on her family's past, Finger's polio-affected protagonist Elizabeth Etters distinguishes "official history" from "that other history," "the things we don't speak of,"[37] suggesting provocative questions: what constitutes official history in this story—the series of leftist causes her parents risked everything to support? The smiling face that any family shows its neighbors, no matter the sadness inside? Which history contains Elizabeth's polio experience? Relative to the alcoholism, abuse, and dysfunction suffered in this family, polio is certainly the least of its shames, yet polio is treated so infrequently, so lightly in this story that it seems indeed to belong to the category of "the things we don't speak of."

Certainly, polio is fitfully on view here: in one instance, Elizabeth dresses for a date in attractive clothes and takes satisfaction from feeling "crippled *and* sexy."[38] In another, she is able to take up tenancy in the rent-controlled apartment vacated by her disabled friend, since "we [crutch-users] all look alike" to the landlady, who indeed fails to notice the difference.[39] Metaphorically speaking, the entire story is about Elizabeth's emotional paralysis, her indecision and inertia with respect to whether to go forward with her pregnancy, her relationship, her career, her life. Yet just as often, polio is a red herring: during a mental breakdown, Elizabeth cuts herself to escape her pain, noting that "at least these are your scars, not the ones the doctors have carved into you" from post-polio corrective surgery.[40] But in fact Elizabeth cuts herself to escape memories of her dysfunctional family, and the reference to polio is largely perfunctory. Overall, as in Sheed's novel, the connection between Elizabeth's polio past and the physical or psychological inhibitions of her present is unclear.

Elizabeth is fascinated, to the point of obsession, by her parents' career as committed, later persecuted leftists and horrified by their later habits of alcoholism and (from her father) paranoia and physical abuse. She hashes over and over her parents' role in the thirties-era radical left, seemingly proud of her father's career in the Abraham Lincoln Brigade fending off the fascists of Spain. She dwells at greater length on her parents' past than on her own; the abuse gets less attention than her red-diaper milieu, and her mid-fifties polio infection is lost within her family's larger crises of persecution and going underground. She is, perhaps more problematically than any protagonist to be read here, crippled by history, yet the narrative fails to work productively with the question of where any individual's true "disability," her actual sources of paralyses, may lie.

Polio at Home

Four novels set in the present consider the polio pasts of main characters whose narrated experience is limited to their circle of family or friends. These stories consider history writ large rarely if at all, recalling only the individual or familial past, and all but one are somewhat in turn limited by this narrow focus and a related, conflicted connection to "history" — inaccuracies regarding polio's own history, stuck-in-the-past attitudes about polio that betray historical unawareness, and lack of a wider context that would make these characters less self-centered and solipsistic. Least troubled on all these counts is Ana Castillo's *Peel My Love Like an Onion* (1999), whose Carmen la Coja is a flamenco dancer who flourishes in American and European cities, but makes the papers (though she is not a historical figure) because she dances on polio-damaged legs. She remarks insightfully upon the simultaneously saved and lost childhood of her demographic, who are removed from harm's way (but also from active life) by polio:

> Here there are babies being born tonight, maybe every night, to babies living for the next killer high—maybe it's bashing in someone's head with a steering-wheel lock, maybe it's sniffing an aerosol can and going into a coma, maybe it's a bullet to the head, bam man it blows everybody's high!
> I never knew this life. The children I went to school with would have been juiced just to wake up with all of their senses intact. What they wouldn't have done to hear, see, think clearly for one day; to get up and walk.[41]

Who, this passage provokes us to ask — between the neglected, mortally threatened street "baby" and the institutionalized, impaired child — is the more disabled by an uncaring society? Who may be said to occupy the upper class in this dichotomy—those free to run the streets long before they are ready for such freedoms, or those clapped into a "private school" that shields them from such dangers yet limits them in every other way as well? In this passage, Castillo partakes of the interesting discussion of polio producing permanent "innocence" yet immediately complicates the question by equating innocence with a sentence to prison. Only in such depressed economic circumstances could health seem an equally demoralizing alternative, and Castillo effectively interimplicates polio and social class.

Carmen's love of flamenco dancing also stems from her specific cultural context, and Castillo creates a productively inverse relationship between flamenco and polio: known for its erotic stylings, flamenco enables Carmen's identity as a desirable woman and unites her with her two main love interests, Manolo and Augustín, who are both connected to the dance world. When post-polio syndrome robs her of her ability to dance, she loses her sexual life as well, as she is abandoned by her lovers in succession. When Carmen is not dancing, therefore, Castillo closes in on what is sometimes a grim reality for women with polio: solitude and sexual unfulfillment. As Carmen ruminates, "Vicky or some other single friend—for some reason it's only single friends who take time to visit lonely women like ourselves . . . might come over with a video. What else should I bring? The friend will ask cheerfully on the phone, and we'll spend the whole time talking while it's playing because I'm not so interested in movies anymore now that I miss my life."[42]

Meanwhile, Castillo reveals a lack of historical awareness in other respects. Most glaring is the strange timing of this novel: Carmen is thirty-six "on the brink of the 21st century"[43] and came down with polio at age six, that is, ten to fifteen years *after* the Salk vaccine. This chronology might have furthered the thesis about social class introduced earlier, that only the most marginalized of children in the United States would be subject to such an avoidable tragedy. Yet Castillo makes no comment on the marked lateness of Carmen's infection, indicating instead her lack of awareness as to the timing of polio's eradication in America and its various stages of manifestation. Such indifference to polio's basic facts suggests a lack of attachment to the illness itself; is polio especially meaningful for this character and her story or simply an interest-generating "crutch"? The question seems pertinent in light of our difficulty imagining Carmen, with one shriveled leg, noticeably shorter than the other, dancing successfully on flamenco stages around the world. How can such a figure, so markedly affected by polio, magically leave her impairment behind in performance? Castillo provides few details, so the effect is impossible to visualize, and Carmen becomes more metaphor or "effect," less a fully realized character.[44] Significantly, Carmen admits that "the memory reels all burn out during my illness and only come back erratically afterward, sporadic frames in which I'm not sure what happened."⁴⁵ The comment reflects Castillo's own lack of memory (historical awareness) during America's own period of polio infection.

The effectiveness of Castillo's depiction of Carmen in her lonely, abandoned situation succeeds very likely because a woman author is thinking critically about the situation of an impaired woman character in a world of men. Perhaps not surprisingly, two male authors depicting polio-affected women fall short of this mark. David Leavitt's Eleanor (*Equal Affections*, 1989) is little more than a caricature, while the condescending handling suffered by Wallace Stegner's Sally (*Crossing to Safety*, 1987) at the hands of her insufferable husband is depressingly typical but not condemned (or even recognized as the abuse it is) by the narrator/author. Leavitt's protagonist, Louise, is seemingly successful—good looks, a stable marriage, a well-appointed home—yet married to a man she never loved and prevented by her own coldness from connecting with her children. Her sister Eleanor is emotionally giving, passionately in love with her husband, and happy in life; she deals successfully with polio's residual effects, while Louise battles recurrent bouts of cancer. As Louise herself concedes, regarding their life-long sisterly competition, Eleanor "had had the upper hand all along."⁴⁶ Yet long ago it was Eleanor's infection from polio, her long convalescence at home, that effectively quarantined the whole family and cut off Louise from Tommy Burns, the dashing love of her youth, consigning her to Nat Cooper, the only boy who came calling outside her window during Eleanor's contagious period. Louise's unhappiness, at least as far is Louise is concerned, is Eleanor's fault.

Leavitt complicates but also reinforces this perspective: he presents Louise's take on the situation as skewed, as a failure to read Tommy Burns as the cad he was and to recognize the value of Nat's devotion, but he never requires Louise to see any of this for herself. To the degree that Louise is an attractive, sympathetic protagonist—and she has many inviting qualities—the reader shares her disdain for Eleanor, her sloppy, off-putting illness and its extremely unfortunate timing. Yet as with Castillo's depiction above, Leavitt's historically inaccurate treatment of polio increases our sense that Eleanor's "crime" is a trumped up charge: she and her family are quarantined for what must have been a considerable period (long enough for Tommy to forget Louise) when in fact the infectious period was never longer than a few weeks, and by this late moment in America's polio era, Eleanor would have been moved immediately to a hospital anyway. Thus Leavitt manipulates the timing of his novel—introducing archaic polio treatment methods into a modern context — to advance the plot and reinforce Eleanor's implication in Louise's life-long unhappiness.

Even as readers see beyond Louise's limited perspective, they are helpless before Eleanor's gross appearance and manner. Somehow, polio must have robbed her of her class status and much of her brain function, for she is slovenly, clownish, and stupid, characteristics she never exhibited in her pre-polio days when she and the beautiful Louise were close. In an introductory scene, Louise "scrutinized her sister who was, as usual, a mess, her hair unwashed and uncombed. She was wearing stretchy pink pants, a blouse with a hideous pattern of yellow flowers, blue sandals through the open ends of which two scratchy blue toenails peeked."[47] Eleanor is too obtuse to recognize how unappreciated her frequent visits to her sister are; she brings homemade pastry that Louise will not eat and sends clippings about the horrors of AIDS — Louise's son is gay — that bring worry, not support. At the hospital during a cancer relapse for Louise, she speaks in condescending pidgin English to a Mexican woman;[48] she and her husband generate part of their income through frivolous lawsuits, and at the end of the story, Eleanor informs Nat that she is suing a computer company for letting its equipment destroy a disk on which she has stored the collection of recipes that enable her main livelihood as writer of a cooking column.

Nat informs her that she has no case, since everyone knows you have to make a back-up disk, yet in fact someone of Eleanor's age and background might not know about the practice of backing up at all. What is truly stupid (i.e., culpable) is Eleanor's burning of the recipes after entering them into the computer. Why didn't she simply throw them out, so that they'd be retrievable when the system crashes the next morning? Because Leavitt would like us to agree with Nat that "that woman is the biggest pain in the ass I have ever known in my life"[49] and to relate this character's physical impairment to her physical unattractiveness and striking stupidity. Nat is furious because no one spared him sitting beside Eleanor at dinner; his son Danny and daughter April are equally disinclined to associate with her, an observation I make to develop a theme introduced earlier: Danny as a contemporary gay man and April as a contemporary lesbian woman are not the "homosexuals" populating the historical fiction I will consider below. While "the pansy" and "the polio" are frequently consigned to each other in these historical narratives, in this modern-day story, Danny and April emerge as fully drawn, interesting characters and join their parents in their disdain for the obnoxious Eleanor.

If we read Eleanor's clownish appearance and foolish behavior as forms of (among other things) infantilizing this female character, Stegner's Sally Morgan is more traditionally feminine and attractive before and after her polio onset and thus infantilized along more traditional lines. In several ways, Stegner's story recalls Mary Grimley Mason's memoir, *Life Prints*, discussed in the previous chapter; both are about privileged academics living "quiet lives."[50] Stegner's is as covertly autobiographical as Mason's is overtly so, and the gender dynamics on display in Mason's story are reflected and reversed in Stegner's. In both stories, the situation of a woman affected by polio is worsened by a domineering husband: in Mason's the woman herself earns the family income and tells the story, while in Stegner's the woman is the dutiful trailing spouse and the narrative object, not subject. Sally's situation seems therefore worse than Mason's, and the notion that her story is "only a novel" is little comfort when so many of the details of Stegner's (and his wife's) own lives have been transposed into the narrative.

Post-polio infection, Sally sits in a "high chair" that Larry is constantly bringing, carrying, and opening for her. The chair "gives her something to push against when she wants to stand again,"[51] yet her husband rescinds this mobility when "with my hands in Sally's armpits I lifted her to her feet."[52] In another scene Larry "gets her established in her high chair" and "spreads [panini] with butter for Sally,"[53] though she is entirely capable of using her arms. "Want to be moved around a little?"[54] he asks another time, reinforcing her post-polio status as total object. At a picnic, she is uncharitably described as offering a toast "from her high chair, looking stiff and incongruous at a luncheon on the grass, but very happy."[55] Sally's "happiness" despite her stiffness and incongruity among these self-important snobs is essential to her depiction as accepting of and even grateful for all her husband does for (and to) her; certainly her willing participation in her own objectification is the most offensive aspect of this character's portrayal: Larry notes that "Sally resented her crutches, . . . but without them she would have been hardly more than a broken stick with eyes,"[56] implanting Larry's cruel observations into Sally's own point of view (her own resentment for her crutches). Perhaps not surprisingly, the most home-bound (and family-centered) of the narratives in this survey focus on female characters with polio; in addition to the many ableist conventions on display, misogynist attitudes (Castillo's characterization notwithstanding) worsen already negative depictions.

Where I critiqued the ahistoric (or unrealistic) handling of polio in these other stories, Howard Owen's *Answers to Lucky* (1996) effectively deploys polio primarily as "effect," a problem that divides family members for decades after its occurrence, even while polio as medical emergency is reduced to mere incident, "the usual horror,"[57] and leaves few residual effects. The story recalls Sheed's novel in both its comic tone and its election-related plot, while it sharply contrasts the family politics on display in Leavitt's novel: in both stories, family members turn against a polio affected character, yet in Owen's the clownish figure of disdain is the father who leads the family in this unconscionable turning-against, while Lucky's having "let down" his family for getting sick years earlier is roundly denounced as bad history. Owen's story is beautifully written, especially its evocation of a special brotherhood—twins bracing in tandem against a demanding, abrasive, even abusive father—that fractures when one boy (ironically, nicknamed "Lucky") is left no more than stiff-legged by polio but is written off as a loss by his success-obsessed father.

What polio has done to worsen an already dysfunctional family dynamic delineates this story's tragic subplot; primarily, it is a fast-moving political comedy about right-wing hypocrisy and southern political hijinks, with Lucky serving as his brother Tom Ed's reluctant but fully capable campaign manager. After a disastrous election and their father's death from the heart attack he fittingly brought on himself, the brothers retreat to Lucky's bed and breakfast in Virginia, where Tom Ed undergoes a physical as well as spiritual recovery: "It's a forty-five minute climb to the top [of the mountain near Lucky's home], although it took Tom Ed an hour and a half the first time Lucky brought him along, while he was still sweating out barbecue and bourbon. But now the twins are in step, on the same pace."[58] Despite their closeness, Lucky is relieved to see his brother return home to his next political bid; as opposed to the clingy, ridiculous Eleanor who never knew when she was not wanted, Lucky is happy outside the limelight, surrounded by his own loving family.

Like Sheed, Owen combines the issues of polio and politics to open similar questions about life's winners and losers, yet unlike Leavitt, Stegner, and several others, he inquires provocatively as to who in the polio-affected family is truly disabled. While polio throughout Owen's novel has not a fraction of the air-time it enjoys in Sheed's striking opening movement, still it persists more successfully as a prevailing theme since it signifies more, and explains more, about the protagonist and his supporting cast from start to finish. Finally, *Answers to Lucky* deals more interestingly with the issues of personal and familial polio history than any of the texts considered thus far: a polio father's inability to let go of the past (his son's moment of infection) traps (we might even say paralyzes) his family at this traumatic juncture even though it is, for all intents and purposes, ancient history. If he is not the worst among the ableist characters in this survey (I would still award Stegner's Larry that dubious distinction) he is likely the most perverse: he insists on seeing a physical disability where it barely exists and is thus, while trapped in a past moment, entirely clueless as to its true magnitude. Polio is thus a metaphor—for dysfunctional paternalism—that ultimately isolates not the polio-affected character but his ableist antagonist.

THE WIDER WORLD

Perhaps not surprisingly, it is during one of his more patronizing caretaking moments in Stegner's novel that Larry makes the insidious pro-Nazi declaration referred to earlier in this chapter: "What if Hitler had broken his pact with Stalin, and German panzers were expanding the war into Poland and Russia? What if the Vichy government of fallen France had just turned military control of Indo-China over to the Japanese?. . . . What if. Forget it. Shoulder the sky, my lad, and drink your ale."[59] This scandalous indifference to history and politics, which defined Stegner's New Critical school of literary analysis and has drawn the ire of more engaged critics in recent decades, reveals here its most morally questionable aspect. All of the remaining novels to be discussed in this chapter open themselves to the obvious significance of history in its various manifestations, even if their success as history or fiction varies markedly.

The four novels I consider in this section broaden their focus from the family and its members to include groups of friends, neighborhoods and towns, and historic happenings on the regional and national scene. Even if the characters in these novels do little traveling themselves, they are affected by national events in significant ways, and a larger sense of history is successfully interwoven with the national and personal narrative of polio itself. As was largely the case in the previous discussion, all of the polio-affected characters here happen to be female; as with Castillo's Carmen, all comment directly or indirectly on the special stigma surrounding the physically impaired woman in able-bodied society. Dorothy Uhnak's *The Ryer Avenue Story* (1993) and Rona Jaffe's *The Road Taken* (2000) look back across the entire twentieth century, replete with crises and triumphs, while Frank Deford's *An American Summer* (2002) and Pat Cunningham Devoto's *My Last Days as Roy Rogers* (1999) both focus on the same summer—the last one before the publication of the Salk vaccine—and depict polio as that season's (and that era's) defining issue.

All four of these novels' central female characters are young, smart, and attractive; only the fourth, Devoto's Tab Rutland, does not herself come down with polio, so will be considered separately later in this discussion. Of the remaining three, Uhnak's Megan Magee is the least physically affected by her illness and happily married by the second half of her story; Jaffe's Ginger Carson uses a wheelchair, is rejected by a boyfriend from Warm Springs and alone but professionally successful at novel's end; Deford's Kathryn Slade is paralyzed from the neck down, uses a respirator for the entire story, and dies in its final pages. The disparity between these women's physical situations and their respective life/love outcomes is grimly realistic, effectively critical, in each case. Plainly, Megan and Ginger have more in common with each other than with the dire Kathryn: both are plucky, privileged New Yorkers, paralyzed only in their lower extremities; both go on to successful careers in medicine. Kathryn is wealthiest of the three, yet her parents' opulent provisions can neither free her from her iron lung nor save her life. Both Megan and Ginger are "fixed up" with homosexuality in the course of their stories; we might say that of the three Kathryn has the most graphic, even unorthodox, sexual experience, yet her death also kills off the possibility of a future romance between this twenty-three-year-old heroine and her loving, deeply devoted, fourteen-year-old friend, Christy Bannister, the story's male protagonist. Even without Kathryn's death, their marked age difference would have been barrier enough to their romance; Deford thus doubly controls against the possibility of his hero Christy having to fall in love with this severely impaired young woman, however beautiful, free-spirited, and fun-loving she may be, or to face the morally unsavory prospect of abandoning her.

Uhnak and Jaffe owe the marked length of their works (400 and 500 pages, respectively) to their epic historical range. In both, polio is but one destination on a whirlwind tour of the American twentieth century: the immigrant waves of the early decades, the world wars, the Depression, the cold war, the sexual revolution, Vietnam, AIDS, gay pride—all the major milestones. Particularly it is Jaffe's explicit project to chronicle the life of a multi-generational family that basically grows up with the twentieth century; Uhnak's focus is on the middle decades, though her story ends in 1970, providing sweeping scope as well. In addition, Uhnak (famous for having written the novel *Law and Order*, whence came the popular TV show) tells a complex crime yarn about a group of tough Bronx junior high-schoolers who take turns clubbing to death the beastly uncle of one of the boys, then pin the job on that same boy's equally beastly dad. How these lives might have suffered (and gained) through the years, in the shadow of this never-confessed "crime"—in fact it was largely self-defense—might have made for an interesting story, but surprisingly, "history" (specifically the polio infection of the tomboy of the group) brings it to a screeching stop. After shifting rapidly from the narrative of one juvenile to the next, as each moves toward then beyond the fateful night of the killing, Megan arrives at camp, succumbs to polio infection, and recovers from her illness in elaborate detail. In fact, Megan's recovery is so complete by novel's end that one hardly remembers her having had polio at all, yet the incident changes the course of the novel: fiction (the interesting crime story) completely gives way to historical subplots—the long polio segment, then various of the main characters in their adult years liberating a Nazi concentration camp, tangling with the Vatican over wartime collaboration, playing a major role in the administration of the early Jewish state, and becoming a senator from New York. In the final pages we return to the (figurative) scene of the crime, as the protagonists confront a blackmailing stool pigeon, but its original mood of fear and excitement has been dissolved.

The structural break (and thematic battle) between fiction and history is not so clear-cut in Jaffe's story. From the beginning, the novel may be seen to suffer from lengthy, pointed digressions into the historical background, and her intent is as clearly to entertain with her story of a complex family as it is to educate with comprehensive overviews. Still, her characters are well drawn; while Megan's polio episode hobbles what had been a fluid, well-paced crime tale, sixteen-year-old Ginger's crisis is a dramatic highlight: "She walked all night, holding on to the walls, to furniture, fighting the pain that was like knives being driven into her leg muscles. As long as I'm upright, . . . she told herself, then I can still walk. . . . At six in the morning, her legs gave way and she fell on the bed, and screamed for her mother."[60] Ginger's more serious impairment and the solitude that results from this continue to dimensionalize her character and the story as a whole; her treatment constitutes a more successful integration of the character and her condition, of fiction and history, than what Uhnak's Megan represents.

Megan becomes active in NOW and writes several articles on women's rights; interestingly, her activism is ascribed not to the sexual revolution of the late '60s but to polio: "do you think, Megan, you'd have gone to medical school and all if, you know, you hadn't gotten polio?" she is asked at one point. "Would you have gotten married right away, right out of high school, like your old pal—Patsy, right? And just settled down to the *normal* life of all the other girls you grew up with?"[61] Here polio functions not only as an aspect of history but as a catalyst for political awareness. Megan's interest in doctoring was largely inspired by her illness, and her braced leg and stigmatized status prevented her from marrying right after high school as most "normal" girls did. The equation between polio, professionalism, and political progressivism is striking here; while many of the most vocal second-wave feminists were those who "made it" in the man's world of work and financial success, Megan might attribute both her professional success and her feminist consciousness to what others might consider her severest limitation—her polio-affected leg.

In striking contrast, Ginger Carson's polio residual is an actual impairment—paraplegia requiring wheelchair use; her success as a medical researcher—and also as a daughter, sister, and friend to many must be measured against her lack of romantic attachment throughout the story. Because Megan married well and had a son, her career and feminism are read as successes. Ginger's equally impressive accomplishments cannot help but function as mere compensations for her many empty nights. If anything, Ginger is depicted as the more interesting, thoughtful, and considerate of the two; she is as beautiful as Megan and reveals to the reader a richer inner life. Yet she is also more polio-affected, and Jaffe deserves credit for facing squarely the disabled woman's all-too-typical solitude instead of contriving a Cinderella ending to salve the reader's guilty conscience.

In what might be deemed another of Uhnak's crime subplots, Megan successfully fends off "accusations" of (and her own self-doubts about) latent lesbianism. Her passionate attachment to fellow-tomboy Patsy in her wild girlhood, strong attitudes on women, and association with the flamboyant Sarah Lawrence student Suzy Ginsberg cause various of the characters to suspect that it is neither polio nor her medical career that almost prevented Megan from being a "normal" girl but her hidden lesbian tendencies. This "charge" is finally dropped, however, since it is the novel's chief antagonist responsible for spreading such bad gossip, while Megan's attachment to her husband and son completes the defense. As a youngster, Megan once confessed to a favorite aunt that she was worried she was one of the "queer girls";[62] after a friendly but intensive third-degree, Aunt Catherine, who is herself sexually unconventional, assures Megan (and us readers) that "You're okay, baby. . . . You're absolutely okay."[63]

Jaffe displays broader-mindedness on this topic, providing readers with not one but two major gay characters and taking them successfully from the closeted early twentieth century through Stonewall, AIDS, and a full-fledged gay rights movement. Yet it is difficult to decide which narrative tactic is more disturbing: Uhnak's clearing Megan of the charge of lesbianism (due to heterosexual success despite polio) or Jaffe's relegation of unmarriageable Ginger to the company of Uncle Hugh and his boyfriend Teddy. Surely it is the outsider status of these three that brings them together time and again; open-minded Ginger accepts her uncle's sexual orientation when her more conservative family members cannot, and when Teddy enters the picture, the three of them are lumped together as an "eccentric triumvirate"[64] who embark on multiple adventures together. It is Ginger's post-polio status that consigns her to the company of the other "sickos" in the family, a thesis reinforced late in the novel when Aunt Daisy, dealing with breast cancer, is cheered by the antics of Hugh and Teddy and spends a holiday party in their company.[65] It is also Ginger's maidenly status that would unite her with the family's "bachelors," though Hugh reminds her at one point that in fact he is happily married to Teddy,[66] making Ginger seem more alone and isolated than ever. Thus neither the "pansies" nor the "polio" seem to benefit from this association, and their "natural" affinity for each other seems to rest on questionable assumptions.

Iron lung-requiring Kathryn Slade, the heroine of Frank Deford's *An American Summer*, stands out among polio-affected characters in this genre for the severity of her physical condition. Deford complicates the portrait by making it plain that her power to function—as friend, mentor, and center of attention—belongs less to her verve and beauty than to her great wealth: the luxury swimming pool her parents have built enables her to preside over neighborhood festivities throughout the summer, and the novel suggests that respirator-requiring youngsters outside such lavish settings would fare much worse. Kathryn is a saddened figure as summer draws to a close, as she knows it will be nine long, chilly months before her "friends" return: yet she asks, "[w]hat good would it do me, to get angry just because people only come to see me because of my pool?"[67] indicating both her serene acceptance of a bad situation and her utter powerlessness to change it. From her bedroom window she bears witness to a climactic event—the rape of her best friend's sister beside that very pool—freeing the girl into the truth of her ultimate innocence even if she can never gain release (physical or sexual) herself.

While Kathryn's role as observer and bearer of truth empower her in certain ways, her reverse peeping-Tom function (she looks out from her action-less bedroom to see sexual activity unfolding on the lawn below) position her as a sexually deprived voyeur, even "pervert." Nancy Mairs has described the discomfort felt by the able-bodied "by the thought of maimed bodies . . . engaged in erotic fantasy or action,"[68] while Susan Wendell observes that "disabled women often do not feel seen (because they are often not seen) by others as whole people, especially not as sexual people."[69] While Kathryn is described, from the neck up, as strikingly beautiful, and while she speaks almost obsessively in graphic terms regarding the sexual attractiveness and interests of the other young people in her purview, her forthright sexuality is a double-edged sword: the novel both calls into question ableist assumptions that those severely affected by polio have no sexual desire and reinscribes the ableist sense that this desire is unnatural (because excessive) and must be punished through ultimate denial of Kathryn's prospects for marriage, childbearing, or sexual fulfillment.[70]

Perhaps influenced (or infected) by his beloved friend's frank manner of speech, fourteen-year-Christy confronts his sister's rapist at a debutante ball by loudly accusing him of "fuck[ing] my sister."[71] The shock of the moment emanates much less from the charge of extramarital sex than from the rough language used to phrase the accusation. Yet it is a red herring: it matters not at all that Sue and Eddie fucked but that she was fucked against her will. In fact, word choice is an issue in this novel pertinent to our understanding of its overall historical accuracy: despite the memorable aspects of Kathryn's polio affliction, Deford seems to get "history" (including the material aspects of polio itself) wrong throughout the story, seriously limiting its value as both a history of polio and a worthwhile fictional work.

Christy and his upper-class, suburban family are a strikingly vulgar bunch, flinging around the "f" word and as noted above engaging in frequent graphic discussions of sex. Kathryn's favorite game is to embarrass Christy with talk of girls' "tits" and to suggest that he is probably a "real ass man"[72] since he does not take enough interest in tits. Was "ass man" even a phrase at this point in history? Was "my ass'll be grass,"[73] "put his ass out to pasture,"[74] "you can take that to the bank,"[75] "blown off,"[76] "that's a crock,"[77] and "that was white of you"?[78] My list is also meant to indicate that despite the shocking crudity of these upper-class characters and their deployment of slang forty years ahead of its currency, they are also untiring dispensers of tiresome clichés: not only do they speak in pat formulas, but their egregiously traditional measures of villainy and heroism—neighborhood toughs running off when a middle-aged man threatens to "tussle with their car,"[79] "noble" Dads sticking to "principles," boys coming of age by winning a backyard swim contest—are also well-worn contrivances instead of authentic situations. These characters' standard-issue '50s-style "innocence" is both utterly incongruous with their crude, anachronistic speech and as unbelievable. Opening the story from the present day, Christy looks back on the history he is about to unfold and declares: "Oh, sure, there were communists. But even as we climbed under our desks for Civil Defense drills, nobody ever seriously considered the possibility that commies might dare actually drop an atomic bomb on us. Come on, get real."[80]

I suggest that it is Deford and his insouciant narrator who need to "get real" regarding the role played by language and history in the story being told. The author's careless handling of the historical detail—he cannot even muster the language to describe skeeball effectively[81]—collides head-on with his ostensible intent to reopen a chapter from the American past. If Deford cannot get the bomb right, can we trust him with the issues of sex, language, and polio itself? Indeed, Deford is frustratingly inconsistent on the details of Kathryn's physical situation. While she sleeps in a full-scale tank respirator, she appears in almost all scenes downstairs by the pool in her portable shell, a device that would fit directly over her chest and leave the rest of her body free. Yet Deford incorrectly pictures Kathryn in some portable version of the tank itself, with her head "emerging" from what is described at one point as "that awful abyss"[82] from which "just her head stick[s] . . . out."[83] In another scene Christy "grabs Kathryn's hand" and falls miserably on his knees, "my head flopping over next to Kathryn's."[84] Finally, all the two can do to give and receive comfort is "touch hair," but if Kathryn's hands are free for the taking, her head would also be clear enough of assistive devices to allow even their cheeks to touch, should Christy position himself appropriately; why does he not? Deford also insists more than once that Kathryn "cannot feel" those who take her hand,[85] yet the paralysis of polio immobilizes but does *not* numb to sensation. Finally, why must Kathryn, after many successful years (six) on respiratory support die at the end of the story? Many respirator users lived long lives inside their tanks, and those who died often did so within the first weeks or months. While certainly some succumbed at this stage in their illness, the timing is too convenient, functioning primarily as a device by which to conclude the summer, the story, and young Christy's obligations to his ultimately burdensome friend.

Like Deford's story, Pat Cunningham Devoto's *My Last Days as Roy Rogers* glows with evocative details from a lost, golden, postwar American moment, and does so for the most part more effectively. While broadly comic stock figures (Tab's grandmother, Maudie's younger brothers) dot the margins of this work, her main characters have interesting conflicts and original personalities; they are strikingly flawed and, most pertinent to this study, put polio to fascinating use. Specifically the juvenile ones use polio as an excuse, a distraction, a means by which to manipulate adults. As was surely the case on countless occasions throughout this period, polio is "in the air" in this circle of family and friends whether it manifests as a headline or personal crisis on any particular day or not. Until the story's final pages, it is just another "polio summer"[86] for young Tabitha, which contains the perennial warnings and fears yet also its share of routine, boredom, and simple pleasures that clash in striking—sometimes incongruous—manner with the mortal threat hanging overhead.

So ingrained into the lived experience is polio for Tab and her community that they refer to the disease as simply "it"; yet the term suggests not only its almost mundane omnipresence but also its terrific, unnameable fearfulness. "To the adults in our world," Tab notes, "it appeared as a giant headlight and they the deer, caught in its beam, afraid to turn in any direction else they or theirs be struck down."[87] Meanwhile, ten-year-old Tab and her high-spirited friends merely chafe at the limitations it brings. In a remarkable scene, Tab's younger brother Charles commences a coughing fit, choking on his dinner. His parents leap up in alarm to feel his forehead for fever, then settle back with relief when they are assured he has no temperature. "[Tab] said, 'Yeah, Charles, you can choke to death all you want to, but just don't get polio. Then you'll really be sorry.'"[88] Here polio has come to obsess Tab's parents to such a degree that they do not even mind their son's choking incident. They deal calmly with what might make other parents hysterical, yet the trade-off is enslavement to the fear that every symptom might mean polio, even false alarms or actual crises (i.e., the choking) that require a completely different response. Even a neighbor's actual death is a relief to Tab's terrorized community: "This was not a polio death. This was a good old all-American heart attack. It was all right to come to the house and not worry about taking home germs. It was all right to visit and talk about it."[89]

For the children, polio threatens to ruin summer by closing down the theaters and swimming pools, yet "it" is a pretty sweet deal in other respects: Tab's neighbor John enjoys a basement full of the best toys, to compensate for his being basically imprisoned there for summer's duration, and when Tom-Sawyerish Tab needs several clay jugs for a fishing expedition, she spins the necessary yarn to free them from her mother's pantry: "J.W.'s mother said drinking a lot of water is one of the things that will help you not get it."[90] When she is about to get into trouble for setting a fire (which in fact she did not set), she "hurries to change the subject": "Say Pop . . . I heard Mr. Peterson got it today. They had to take him to the hospital."[91] Early in the story, polio is even, ironically, a free ticket to the movies for Tab and her fellow girl scouts. They pass March of Dimes collection boxes at the end of the program and are allowed to attend for free, right before the theater closes for the summer. Thus, despite the deer-in-the-headlights paralysis it induces at one level, polio frees several of the story's characters (especially the younger ones) for more autonomy and adventure than they might otherwise enjoy.

The theater in this small southern town is an emblem of another of the novel's major themes—the racial segregation that divides black and white townsfolk (and even Tab's politically mixed family) in the fifties-era South. Passing her coin box through the rows of the main floor, Tab spies her new friend, Maudie May, in the balcony and notes with envy that the black filmgoers of Bainbridge, Alabama are freed from the policing ushers and, on this day, the antics of the coin collectors below. When various of Tab's white friends start climbing over the seats and creating chaos, "March of Dimes canisters became footballs spiraling through the air, spraying coins as they sailed."[92] So much for the good works of Tab and her friends, despite Tab's own emotional reaction to a March of Dimes promotional reel, featuring a man in an iron lung thanking the theater audience for its support. Here Devoto effectively associates a failure, however small, on the polio homefront with a backward, segregationist mindset; in this scene, the black patrons are both intellectually and physically superior to the white hijinks transpiring below, and the theater seems the setting for all-around bad behavior—childishness, racial discrimination, lost funds for polio. Not only does the closing theater (and, for that matter, the likewise-segregated swimming pool) protect from potential polio contagion; it frees the citizens of Bainbridge from their falsely divided seating arrangements, enabling the inter-racial friendship of Tab and Maudie May to blossom over the summer.

Together the girls build a secluded fort in the remote, even dangerous part of the woods; bowered thus, they imagine that "if the whole town came down with polio and half the people were dead . . . we might have to come here and live for ever and ever."[93] To keep away outsiders, the girls select an off-putting name, perhaps not surprisingly by now, "Fort Polio," though narratively speaking, the choice does not work: in fact, this setting is a vital escape for the girls and to name their secret hiding place after that which they are primarily hiding from is implausible. In sentences that jangle strangely—"We had pretty much settled into a routine at Fort Polio"[94] and "of everybody in this here Fort Polio, who is the best reader?"[95]—this incongruity is even more pronounced. When Tab flees a difficult scene at home one day—"Straight to Fort Polio, the place I felt most comfortable now"[96]—the term seems to have lost most of its fearfulness, that is, its specificity, meaning, and history.

Devoto sends her girl heroines on a thrilling fishing trip downriver, invoking Huck Finn's story as well as Tom Sawyer's, demonstrating the ways in which strong, bright Maudie May has left the troubling aspects of Jim's character behind. When at last it is Maudie May who succumbs to polio at novel's end, Devoto would critique the patterns of segregation that reassert themselves when "it" moves from hovering threat to actual occurrence: confined to the balcony of the theater in nonepidemic times, Maudie is sent off to the hospital for Negroes when she takes sick, then even farther away to Tuskegee's rehabilitation center, excising her from Tab's orbit and the story itself. In one respect, Devoto creates an analogy between race and disability "inscribed by history" (i.e., segregated rehabilitation facilities in pre-Civil Rights America) in a manner similar to that read by Rosemarie Garland Thomson in the fiction of African-American women writers. Thomson argues that in these works, the black female characters are "marked" not so much by their racial or bodily particularities as by historical forces that see and position them to their disadvantage.[97] Lennard J. Davis also sees a parallel between race and disability, two cultural constructs activated by the dominant culture's substitution of a continuum (occupied by degrees of skin pigmentation, physical abilities, etc.) with a permanent is/is-not divide.[98] In Devoto's story the divide is literal and politicized: like Thomson's "history," polio "marks" Maudie May as not only sick (contagious) and disabled but also, once more, as "black," requiring rehabilitation in segregated, perhaps underfunded facilities in the story's off-stage environs.

The antisegregation message is clearly sent in this writing, yet the narrative movement here is identical to that which concludes Deford's novel, which I questioned above and question here for the same reasons: in Devoto's story, racism is as overwhelming a factor as is death for Deford; as Christy moves blamelessly into the future freed of his ties to the severely impaired Kathryn, here Tab returns to her (all-white) school and her middle-class life without the complicating factor of Maudie May's friendship. In later years she is comforted by rumors of her friend's success as a feisty fish camp operator in another part of the state, yet such an upbeat scenario conflicts with the possibility that Maudie May "died on the train headed for Tuskegee,"[99] (355), neither of which is Tab ever able to verify.[100] Tab concludes her story with a happy recollection of her past days with Maudie May—dancing under the water pouring off her roof after a rain[101]—but what about their present and future as friends? Tab's racial privilege enables her to put polio and all this term has come to stand for into her own bittersweet past, but for the less fortunate Maudie, polio is either her permanent present or perhaps, simply, her end. Again, this turn of events makes for a dramatic ending, but the novel is almost as comfortable leaving behind Maudie May for her race as for her disability.

Both Deford's and Devoto's novels, then, effectively reconstruct a moment in American history through deployment of polio as their most evocative theme; in both, however, the abandonment of the polio-affected character by the able-bodied protagonist (i.e., by the narrative itself) not only uncritically mirrors the incidence of such leave-takings throughout American history, even to the present day, but serves the ideological mandate of mainstream fiction as well: despite its tragic dimension, the death or disappearance of the polio-affected character enables happy endings for the unscathed protagonist and his or her able-bodied readership as well. Disability theorist Paul K. Longmore has critiqued such fortuitous plot turns—depressingly recurrent in stories with disabled characters—for "allow[ing] the nondisabled audience to disown its anxieties and prejudices about disabled people."[102] Thus, as the protagonists of both these novels are granted eleventh-hour access to the moral high ground, so the reader finds absolution for her own ableist presumptions regarding the "life worth living." In forcing their polio-affected heroines into permanent states of innocence (in their untouchable disabilities and in their early, angelic deaths), these novels make the only move that can confer innocence upon their lead characters and readers as well.

History Writ Large

Four novels whose integration of history (polio and other major events from the American twentieth century) with fiction is especially complex and rewarding will constitute a final analytic grouping in this chapter. Each may be critiqued for its placement of polio within the narrative— either saving its polio-affected character for a big finish or leaving him behind in the narrative sweep toward climax and resolution—yet each integrates the polio theme, even if only metaphorically, in meaningful ways by expanding its significance into philosophic and world-political registers. Possibly related to each story's wider reach is its gendering of plot and characters as primarily masculine: in each, a male polio-affected character is part of a larger mostly male community engaging in masculine leisure, work, and military pursuits. Meanwhile, as per the arguments made at the beginning of this chapter, the polio-affected boys in each story remain boys or are infantilized by their texts in ways that disable, disempower, even feminize their characters. Tony Earley's *Jim the Boy* (2000) and Michael Köepf's *The Fisherman's Son* (1998) are stories of bygone eras rooted in an ambiguous past, presenting endearing boy protagonists in peaceful, coastal outposts of U.S. society. Jim is a "town boy" in rural South Carolina and Köepf's Neil is the son of a commercial fisherman in the Pacific Northwest. Jim's father dies shortly before Jim is born, but he is raised by three uncles and his loving mother; aside from his mother, with whom he does not connect, Neil knows only men and boys from the hardscrabble fishing community that draws him into its traditions. Both boys have a friend with polio: the illness and paralysis of Jim's friend Penn Carson is "saved" for the end and enables Jim to come of age; similarly, Billy "the Raisin" Bergstrom is a wheelchair-using background figure throughout Neil's story who plays a major role in the story's final pages. In both, polio functions as the marker of "history" to the degree that it represents the decline and passing of an idyllic age, the very phenomenon of change itself, introduced into a timeless, elemental environment. In Earley's story, Penn's frightening brush with polio signals the death of Jim's innocence (even as Penn is now trapped forever in dependent boyhood), while Köepf's polio-affected character "anchors" the other sailors in his group so as to save their lives.

In Earley's lyrical, evocative tale friendship grows between Jim and Penn (a mountain boy), who comes down with polio during an argument about who will use a baseball glove. Practically forced to visit Penn during his convalescent period, Jim leaves him the glove out of both regard and guilt. Tragically, Penn's illness has left him as worn down as the decrepit, malevolent grandfather Jim sees for the first time during this same trip up the mountain: the boy falls asleep shortly after Jim arrives, their game of catch called to an abrupt halt, and the reader is as shaken as is Jim by the obvious fragility of Penn's health and perhaps chance for survival. His new lack of mobility reflects the sense of being trapped that Jim has always associated with mountain people. He feels fortunate to have escaped his mountain roots but during his visit is surprised to learn that Penn's cultured mother, who has seen Philadelphia and New York, is actually happily settled in her mountain home — a surprisingly spacious, comfortable-seeming place. In addition, Jim is awed by the view from so high up, a perspective that contrasts with his long-held sense of mountain people as narrow-minded and impervious to change. It is this mountain view that causes Jim to realize that "there was nothing he could do inside that circle [his town's layout on view below] that would matter much to anyone outside it."[103] In the midst of a changing world, signified by Jim's own changing perception of the alien backwardness of mountain life, Penn's polio represents an equation between mountain culture and permanent entrapment associated with outdated perceptions. It exemplifies a past that everyone in the story understands he must move beyond, painful as that transition might be. Penn's inability to come down the mountain, perhaps ever again, has caused Jim to make a climb that prevents him from returning to town as his old self. When he insists at story's end that he is still "just a boy,"[104] his uncles remind him, "But you're *our* boy,"[105] seeming to throw down the challenge that he use the lessons of the day to make full use of his own mobility, even if it means eventually stepping beyond the circle.

If the boys' stories of Twain are distant forerunners of Earley's work, the tradition of Hemingway may be recognized beneath the waves of Köepf's gripping yarn of men battling an always eventually triumphant sea. Neil's father and fellow-fisherman ply an ancient trade whose methods are just beginning to modernize during Neil's boyhood. While technology makes fishing easier, corrupt wholesalers demand a greater percentage of profits with each passing year, exacerbating seasons of bad catches that have been part of the fisherman's cyclical temporal experience for centuries. Now, Neil's community "was changing too. Different people were coming, spilling over the hills from the suburbs, people who didn't grow artichokes or own a fishing boat. . . . [P]eople you did not know and who did not want to know you."[106] The narrative itself fights the encroachment of history by telling a primarily timeless tale; rare are the temporal references that would locate this story in any particular decade (or century). When Neil's brother makes an excited reference to "commie torpedoes,"[107] the reader is jarred into historical locatedness for the first time, as when a ship runs aground. Later references to a wealthy president, his striking wife, his eventual assassination, anchor the story even more specifically in the "post-vaccine" phase of the postwar era, though certainly the presence of "the Raisin" with his wheelchair and withered limbs sets the story well within the lingering polio period.

Despite the troubling changes faced by Neil's community as history rushes coastward to embrace and engulf it, the narrative also depicts Neil's father, his friends, and the sons who are pulled, even unwillingly, toward the fishing life in their fathers' wake as dangerously "at sea," and searches for anchors to save them. While Neil contemplates "the world beyond Half Moon Bay" and wonders "whether it was worth going there,"[108] he also feels himself merely "drifting into the future" of a life at sea,[109] instead of consciously choosing such. His mother, sensibly aware of the mortal dangers and financial hardships belonging to the profession, begs him to consider other options. By contrast, the markedly impaired Raisin is in love with the sea-faring life and longs to succeed as a one-armed, wheelchair-using commercial fisherman, though he has never been in a boat before he is spirited away by the other boys one fateful afternoon. I read this polio-affected character as an envoy of "history," whose first contact with what lies outside history—the sea itself—is a collision resulting in near tragedy. Encountering rough water, the boys' boat is deluged, with oars, motor, and provisions tumbling overboard. As freezing night sets in, the boys drift farther from shore; only when the Raisin realizes that his wheelchair can be flung from the boat on a line and anchored among the rocks below can the boys arrest their movement until morning, when their fathers' boats find and save them. Significantly, the line connecting the chair ("history") to the rocks of the sea ("a-history" or "fiction") is "not much better than string,"[110] suggesting that the anchoring of "the timeless" to the historical is as simple as it is tenuous: change brings the opportunity that may free Neil (or perhaps his own children) into an easier life yet also suggests that even the Raisin might succeed in this strenuous work environment if he can use modern methods to connect him to support and safety.

If Earley and Koëpf involve polio characters in novels that address large philosophical questions regarding the human perception of time's passing, the encroachment of time into space, large historical questions are revisited and productively engaged with the issue of polio in two political thrillers set in the middle twentieth century: Michael Chabon's *The Amazing Adventures of Kavalier and Clay* (2000) and James Carroll's *Secret Father* (2003). In contrast to the novels by Earley and Koëpf, and by

Uhnak, Jaffe, Deford, and Devoto, all of which focus their action in the homes and neighborhoods of family members and friends involved for the most part in local actions, the polio-protagonists of Chabon's and Carroll's novels are young men in world cities who bear witness to momentous historical events and live active, unencumbered lives: Chabon's Sammy Clay is a talented New York comic book artist who teams with his Czech-born, Nazi-fleeing cousin to turn the tide of American isolationism through their revolutionary comics; Carroll's Michael Montgomery is a high school student in early-sixties West Germany who makes a fateful trip East with two idealistic friends just as the Wall threatens to permanently prohibit their return. Significantly, Chabon's and Carroll's texts circumvent the "age of innocence" (the 1950s), so lovingly excavated in, for instance, Deford's and Devoto's novels; their respective World War II and Cold War contexts raise the stakes all around, yet their larger historical canvases threaten, and in fact supplant, the centrality of polio as a theme, as is not the case with Deford's and Devoto's poliocentric works. That polio continues to thematically inform and enrich even those stories that attempt in certain ways to leave it behind speaks to its power as a textual and subtextual element in contemporary novelistic treatments of the past. Meanwhile, it is perhaps even less surprising (though no less disappointing) that the action-packed plotlines and epic sweep of these latter novels ultimately sideline their polio-affected characters, as do many of the other novels in this survey.

In Chabon's story, it is not our hero Joseph Kavalier but his cousin and sidekick Sammy Clay who is affected by polio, while Carroll's protagonist Michael is the brace- and cane-using son of an executive working in postwar Germany just as Berlin splits traumatically into East and West. In both stories, the themes of "escape" and "flight" (as in "fleeing to the West") resonate effectively with the hobbled conditions of their lead characters; it is Michael who looks at East Germany and thinks of it as "crippled by history" (whence comes this chapter's title), while it is he who must escape its rapidly closing borders in time and may not be physically up for the challenge. Finally, despite their many strengths, both stories lose a specifically political (and thrilling) momentum as they move toward conclusion. Chabon's gripping account of a young Jewish man's escape from Nazi Czechoslovakia gives way to the perforce less urgent narrative of his life in the States as a comic book artist, while Carroll's story stays focused on political intrigue but loses steam by overly slow pacing at novel's end. In each case, the attempt to fill such a large historical canvas results in a complex, uneven structure that interestingly replicates the experience of polio itself—crisis at the outset, winding down to staid routine—yet might have forged a stronger connection to polio to maintain dramatic tension and to enrich the relationship of each novel to the past it attempts to rejuvenate.

With respect to direct references, Sammy's polio is in fact a fairly extraneous feature in Chabon's six hundred-page story. His legs jiggle when he is nervous, a word or two is provided as to their thinness, and he is diffident around the opposite sex. When he first encounters Rosa, who later falls in love with Joe, she asks "is he a fairy?"[111] when she notes his anxious desire to escape her company. At this point Sammy—who *is* gay—has not come out (even to himself), so that the more accurate response to her question would be, "no, he just has polio." His condition keeps him out of the draft and out of participation in social activities—swing dancing, parties, dates; his passion for comics absorbs him in the environment of Charles Atlas and other quick fixes for scrawny kids on sale in the comics' fine print, and he figures throughout the narrative as the eternal kid and classic ninety-eight-pound weakling. Despite the fact that Sammy's (note even his youthful, unserious name) irrepressible humor and energy in part undermine the notion of polio as a depressing or enfeebling condition, his infantilization, as I observed above, has its problematic qualities from a disability-studies standpoint. Likewise, queer studies has challenged the infantilizing, the Freudian-style pathologizing, of gay and lesbian identities as cases of arrested development. Robert McRuer discerns the parallel systems by which heterosexuality and able-bodiedness are normalized by the hegemonic mainstream: the consolidation of queerness and disability "occurs through complex processes of conflation and stereotype: people with disabilities are often understood as somehow queer . . . , while queers are often understood as somehow disabled."[112] The mainstream's habit of pathologizing disabled sexuality (discussed above) corroborates McRuer's argument. In Chabon's novel, Sammy is less doubly or simultaneously than serially oppressed: his gay identity surfaces once his polio identity recedes, yet both remove him from the action of heterosexual and military conquest—two of the story's main preoccupations.

Specifically, Sammy's physical condition bears not at all on his abilities as an artist, writer, deal-maker, and ground-breaker in the comics industry; he gets his best story ideas—and has a life-changing encounter with his itinerant father—on lengthy, arduous walks through New York City, never needing to rest. He shares a romance with an attractive man, marries his beloved friend Rosa when Joe disappears during the war, and raises Joe and Rosa's son; his ultimate lack of sexual fulfillment and later professional decline are *both* more attributable to his homosexuality than to polio[113] and the sporadic references to it in this sprawling story function less as a complete subplot than as a mere reminder that Sammy has polio at all.

And yet polio resonates wonderfully with so many of the novel's more essential themes. Movement and mobility are of course vital to young Joe in the course of his harrowing flight from Nazi-threatened Prague. As a boy, he admired the skills of Harry Houdini and learned the art of escape from a local eccentric. His facility for the craft enables him to flee Hitler's clutches, but he has left behind his parents and younger brother and is consumed with the effort to save them. When he ultimately fails in this attempt, he flees once again, into the US army to join the battle against the Germans, where he again performs daring feats. The cartoon he and Sammy invent is the Escapist, a Hitler superfoe whose humble alter-ego is Tom Mayflower, who himself relies on a crutch for mobility, and transforms into a superhero with the help of a golden key. One of the cousins' fellow-comic artists observes that comics are about "Wishful figments. You know, like it's all what some little kid *wishes* he could do. Like for you [Sammy], hey, you don't want to have a gimpy leg no more. So, boom, you give your guy a magic key and he can walk."[114]

And not only walk, of course. In classic comics style, the Escapist's physical acts are fantastically superhuman, suggesting that Sammy's dreams for physical mobility are far-reaching—he himself, for instance, might wish to battle Hitler's armies in uniform instead of ink—and ultimately impossible to attain. While the novel may lament Sammy's limitation and do its best to compensate by providing him with a successfully executed mission (the anti-Hitler comics series) of his own, in fact it is his able-bodied cousin Joe who has all of the "amazing adventures" in the story, while Sammy, despite the relatively minor nature of his polio impairment, is bound to the home front and lives a comparatively ordinary life.

It is not Hitler but Stalin, and the deadly politics of his communist empire, that ground the actions of a polio-affected character, his friends, and their worried parents in Carroll's *Secret Father*. The ability to move quickly, even flee surreptitiously, is as important a skill in the fraught context of early-sixties Berlin as it was in Nazi-threatened Prague twenty years earlier, though Carroll raises Chabon's stakes to the degree that he places a polio-hobbled young American in the company of two other shortsighted teenagers who find themselves trapped in East Berlin just as the iron curtain is descending in this region of Europe. Michael's father Paul refers to his son as an innocent "bystander,"[115] a term that rings with irony when pages later he critiques for "that famous bystander detachment"[116] the Germans who acquiesced throughout the war, and when we recall that Michael can barely stand at all: in fact Michael is much more involved (and perhaps much guiltier) than his father may understand or acknowledge; as with the parents of many polio-affected children in polio novels, Paul's sense that polio will keep his son "innocent" (unable to fend for himself or to create trouble) must be thoroughly revised in the course of the story.

Michael's use of cane and braces does not prevent him from joining his friends, the charismatic Ulrich and fetching Kit, on a political pilgrimage to the revolutionary East. Ulrich is a zealous socialist, disdainful of his high school's athletes and cheerleaders, who persuades his friends to join him for the May Day festivities. Michael himself is of course an outcast in the West's cult of beauty, whose recent manifestation as Hitler's brutal policy of eugenics meant that "Cripples like [Michael] had been gassed."[117] While he is much less the fanatic than Ulrich, he recognizes, as the Eastern countryside rumbles past the windows of their train, a kindred spirit in the largely failing project of rebuilding humbly from the rubble of war:

> I had seen the East as a truncated nation on the losing side of history. Shot by history—no, crippled by history. I myself was no gleaming city alight with beauty, no polished locomotive—no true rebel either, on an authentic quest. What I had seen looking out the train window was a world improperly aligned with itself....
>
> But that wasn't all I had seen. I had caught glimpses of my own reflection, wild flashes of disconnection there as well.[118]

Meanwhile, Michael has already noted that even Ulrich's socialist idol Marcuse cannot promise "freedom from crutches,"[119] reinforcing once more Michael's status as "innocent bystander"—pulled into this dangerous journey by his forceful friend, yet ultimately excluded from the dream Ulrich hopes to realize at the end of it. More than anything, Michael is "running from"[120] what countless "normal" boys have sought to escape—the suffocating reach of his overprotective father, who insulted Michael's masculinity by suggesting he major in fine arts in college (among other atrocities) and is therefore largely responsible for the fix Michael gets into.

The three youngsters move with ease from West to East (the freer direction of travel in this period), despite their moving against an enormous tide of refugees going in the opposite direction while the going is still good. Once a roll of film, stowed inadvertently in Ulrich's bag, calls them to the attention of the authorities, their movement grinds to a halt, and Michael's impairment becomes a pronounced issue: his cane is taken from him during a confrontation with the police, and he is forced to "lope along with an exaggerated stride"[121] when the three are moved from one holding area to another. He realizes that he threatens the escape all three may be forced to make if their parents cannot free them through the proper channels.[122] Their particular historical context intensifies the crisis: as difficult as it may be to flee an authoritarian regime by crossing a forbidden border, imagine scaling a wall and dropping safely to the other side with two heavy braces and paralyzed legs.

Despite these high-stakes possibilities, the stories' conclusion stumbles in a welter of names, roles, secret pasts, political associations, and moral positionings. Like Michael's own brace-without-cane situation, historical weight hobbles the movement of the fictional narrative when the great secret that would explain the specific trouble the kids are in is withheld at length then disappointing once revealed. The shocking revelation includes the possibility that Ulrich's mother, Charlotte, used to be a communist, but in 2003, when this story was published, the reader hardly cares. Once it would have been a disturbing fact; today, for better or worse, it is "ancient history" and fails as a piece of authentic intrigue. In its final chapters, the story reverts curiously to the actions and mis/perceptions of the teenagers' parents; not only do their comparatively square doings and discoveries weaken narrative interest, but the story thus reverses its coming-of-age thematic by suspending action for (i.e., paralyzing) all three youngsters, who wait off stage for their middle-aged forebears to rescue them. When we recall that one of these three young people is literally paralyzed, the narrative's infantilizing gesture is unfortunately not so curious at all. In the book's epilogue, the main characters reunite decades later to witness the collapse of the Wall. Here we are subjected to lengthy overviews of the rise and fall of communism between '61 and '89; even Michael, listening to his father speak, feels "he recited a narrative as if he had rehearsed it. . . . I felt as if I were hearing the voice-over of a Cold War documentary."[123] Intrigue thus gives way to academic meditations from the secure ineffectuality of the post-Wall narrative present, the parental voice forcefully, however tediously, predominating.

Even as both Chabon's and Carroll's recurring themes of movement, flight, and escape enable such a productive conceptual interchange between polio and the politics that defined the middle twentieth century, their very focus on these concepts ensures that Sammy and Michael will be eventually sidelined by their own storylines—that they are destined to function only tangentially in their literal polio-affectedness, while the metaphoric significance of their condition travels the larger narrative without them. Their respective "wishful figments" of action and heroism are to be enacted by their able-bodied advocates, as neither youth is ever put to the physical test. We might observe that a polio-affected character with leg weakness or braces cannot fight German soldiers or scale the Berlin Wall any more plausibly than s/he can flamenco-dance to world acclaim; as Michael Köepf has shown, however, action plots *can* be constructed that effectively, centrally involve a polio-affected character; while his "small" story lacks the impressive sweep of Chabon's and Carroll's, the polio affecting his unassuming hero, "the Raisin," is both a powerful metaphor (for the encroachment of time, for history itself) and a realistically deployed, essential aspect of the boy's distinctiveness and heroism.

As sweeping and complex as they are, major historical conflicts of the kind featured centrally in these novels by Chabon and Carroll call into question the moral claims to innocent-bystanderism, made even (or especially) by the able-bodied who witness and do nothing. An implicit thesis of both novels, then, is that action against tyranny is the only moral gesture, yet both novelists place their polio-affected protagonists in the vicinity of heroic action, then sideline them for lack of faith in their physical abilities. By their limitations, both Sammy and Michael are proclaimed "innocent" of failing to act, yet the proclamation is a false one; the level of ability exhibited by both could have enabled much more active, heroic roles. While many of these novels may be congratulated for calling into question the innocence of the American mid-century, they must be faulted for failing to question the ableist attitudes of that period, which kept physically impaired persons (and story characters) confined to states of limited, impotent innocence—a failure that perpetuates these attitudes into the present day.

Postscript: The Future of Polio

What are certainly the two most widely read and best sold novels in this survey—James Patterson's *Cradle and All* (2000) and Stephen Coonts's

Cuba (1999) — both take the intriguing step of catapulting polio (in Coonts's case, literally) into the future, when my focus throughout has been on polio's relationship to the past. As has been the case with all the texts considered here, these use history (i.e., historical figures) to temporally situate the reader, but in both cases, the situation is not the postwar past but some undefined point in the near future: in Patterson's story, "Pope Pius XIII" presides inconsequentially over a farfetched contest between God and the Devil, while Coonts's context is the last days of Castro and the power struggle that ensues upon his death. Like Patterson's, Coonts's novel has its fantasy elements: America dreams of the day when Castro's era will finally end, when America will happily reoccupy charming Havana and exploit Cuba's cheap labor markets, and when its weapons of war (aimed at Cuba or elsewhere) will achieve the surgical precision Coonts zealously depicts. While I could list at length the many reasons why I feel these stories fail as both fiction and (especially) history, a prominent culprit is both stories' unsuccessful attempt to locate polio at a moment in America's future, when its imbrication in the past will always be the more productive object of literary exploration.

Polio is in fact a side issue in both novels. In *Cradle and All*, the death of countless children from "the old menace with a new, more potent kick"[124] heralds the advent of the Devil on earth, then recedes with a host of other disasters — "famine in India . . . plague in Asia"[125] — when the story's protagonists complete their heroic quests. At novel's end, a heroic priest takes the devil child over a high cliff into the sea with him, and "children with polio stopped arriving in hospitals";[126] whether the virus will handily re-emerge when "a boy who'd been thrown from the cold Irish Sea and survived"[127] returns to wreck havoc in the sequel is a question only Patterson's more devoted readers will have the answer to.

In Coonts's story, yet another super-charged strain of polio has been concocted to fill the warheads of Cuban missiles aimed at the southeast United States. While the virus is so rapidly malignant that it looks nothing like polio — an infected victim is folded in half backwards within seconds[128] — in fact polio is a clever choice on this author's part, a bogey from America's postwar past that, like Cuba, no longer scares us. Like Cuba, polio was stopped in its tracks in the mid-twentieth century and effectively evokes present-day Cuba's fifties-era look — its "vintage" cars, streets, and buildings that charm American outsiders but also signify Cuba's long era of economic paralysis and surely somewhat depress Cubans themselves. Visiting modern Cuba is stepping back into the past; revisiting American fear of Cuba (and polio) through revival of the 1960s showdown constitutes a walk down memory lane that Coonts's warring patriots risk their lives to avoid taking. The fire set by the story's protagonists to destroy the virus lab works magically, achieving just the right degree of heat to destroy the entire plant yet not spread the super-strain in any sort of overheated explosion.

Coonts's alter-ego, Navy hero Jake Grafton, observes that biological weapons are both "deadliest" and "cheapest," making them especially tempting to "Third World" countries[129] such as Cuba, who seek America's attention. While another author might turn such an observation toward the case for improving the situations of and relations with the developing world, Coonts's military commanders advise the president to sign treaties then ignore them.[130] If such dialogue sounds less like murmurings from the dark ages or fantastic futurism than business as usual with respect to present-day US foreign policy, the novel returns to the register of right-wing fantasy in its final pages, when a CIA operative tracks down and blows away the mad scientist who concocted the superstrain in the first place: he is an American (could the "Third World" produce a scientist smart enough?) but a crazed academic from the liberal bastion of Boulder, Colorado.

Conclusion

If both Coonts and Patterson get polio wrong by exaggerating its physical effects, most of the other novels in this chapter do so by underplaying either the parameters of its limitations or its grim finalities. Departing from theorists who read disability metaphors in a negative light,[131] I applaud novels that embed the issue of polio in larger historical narratives by exploring the conceptual similarities between polio and war, polio and politics, polio and the American past. Meanwhile, in accordance with these and other disability theorists, I reject novelistic attempts that confine polio-affected characters themselves to the narrative margins, to an enforced childhood that alienates them from their come-of-age historical contexts, or that treat their conditions in a fanciful or overdramatized (historically inaccurate) manner. Even as the historical revisions often contained in polio novels call into question the middle twentieth century as an American era of innocence *and* explore the frustrating prohibitions against coming of age experienced by their polio-affected characters, these novels undo this work to the degree they themselves infantilize these characters by removing them from the main action. In all of the novels considered here, polio's shift from the heart of narrative significance to the thematic and plot-driven margins indicates each text's own shift from realism to romance, from historical accuracy to "mere" metaphor, from (individual) childhood trauma to (national) childhood innocence, from remembering to forgetting the polio past.

Interestingly, all but three of the novels considered in this chapter have been published since 1993, with about one-third debuting in the last half-dozen years. As I have implied throughout this chapter, timing is everything: the nonfiction texts, especially those issuing from polio's own "present," were a natural initial reaction to the crisis. Now (and perhaps only now) that polio is in several respects "over"—and thus now that polio is in danger of being forgotten by historically amnesiac American readers (especially, the youngest of these)—have novelists joined the fray. The historical novelist may seek to educate or to obfuscate, may do one as s/he attempts the other, and in this case may take up the theme of polio so as to explore (or exploit) its own significance or that which relates it to other once-terrifying contexts and questions from the American past. I hope to have shown that this historically informed longer view, with all the insight its critical distance affords, must also guard against an accompanying emotional distancing that will undermine any novel as both literature and history.

4

"Heads, You Win!": Newsletters and Magazines of the Polio Nation

IN MAY 1961 THE FOUNDING EDITORS OF THE *TOOMEY J. GAZETTE*, WHICH began as a newsletter for a respiratory polio clinic in Cleveland and became an internationally circulated magazine, wrote a four-page letter to the Department of Health, Education, and Welfare, pleading for the lives of people with respiratory polio. This population of severely impaired Americans was about to lose its vital sources of funding, treatment, and personal care attendance, as the National Foundation for Infantile Paralysis wound down its operations nationwide due to a sharp decline in contributions—and the national perception that the polio problem was "over"—following the Salk vaccine in 1955. The editors, Sue Williams, who was herself an iron-lung user, and Gini Laurie, who lost three siblings to polio and was dubbed late in life "the grandmother of the independent living movement,"[1] described with eloquence the persisting presence of this group in the American midst: "We are Chronic Respiratory Polios—occupants of iron lungs or their equivalents. We are new world of people."[2]

This new world, or new nation if you will, was a singular product of its moment in time: pre-vaccine, in that those with respiratory polio became infected and paralyzed before the vaccine was available, but, as the editors imply, were post-antibiotics and other supportive medicines, which by the early 1960s saved many such fragile lives that might have been otherwise lost. They were post-polio—safely past its most life-threatening stages—but not at all done with its lasting effects, as more fortunate Americans felt themselves to be by the early 1960s. They were, in contrast to a forward-looking, ever-healthier American society, stuck in a pre-vaccine past, and as is the case with all veterans of tragic, concluded wars, on the verge of being forgotten by the mainstream. It was up to the editors to convince the government that, like this American mainstream, "we are young, energetic, and healthy (Yes! Healthy!)," that "we ["respiratory polios"] have our brains, and we are capable of running our homes and earning a living."[3] Williams and Laurie described women and men in their prime struck down—not by polio but by lack of financial support—leaving families floundering, separated, and sent into foster care. The vigorous rhetoric and vital message on display in this appeal matches the approach taken in the editors' regularly appearing *Gazette*, where Laurie would later forthrightly engage with her beloved community of "heads" in an editorial whose title is my own.

The *Gazette* produced by Williams and Laurie, as well as multiple other newsletters and inter/national magazines published during the early postwar/polio rehab era in the United States, exemplify the vitality and political significance of the recovering polio community itself, much of which would form the first population of Americans with physical impairments to lobby successfully for disability rights. These typed, mimeographed, stapled, and freely circulated sheets and booklets aided recovering "polios" (a term they themselves used, irreverently and subversively) in the formation of communal and individual identities. These were identities that successfully included their illness and impairment experiences, even as those waiting for them to return to able-bodied productivity sought to deny and minimize this new reality. While polio publications took many forms, some nearly indistinguishable from any general interest magazine, many "embodied" the polio experience for their readership by situating the body plainly, productively, and with spirited wit in the center of the writing and reading experience.

Like the mass-marketed polio memoirs discussed earlier in this study, the rehab center ephemera and specially published magazines under consideration in this chapter take the reader into the heart of the polio experience. As opposed to postwar-era women's magazines, which situated its readership specifically but safely *before* the terrifying reality of polio, and as opposed to recently published polio novels whose audience encounters these texts many eventful decades *after* the end of the polio era in America, both memoirs and newsletters are *intra*-polio genres, whose *raison d'etre* is the onset of and multidimensional adjustment to polio illness and impairment. The newsletter, however, differs importantly from the memoir in its handling of its crisis and denouement: while the memoir is a singular text with a definite conclusion, which almost always concludes its narrative by leaving polio behind, the serial form constituting the newsletter or magazine is best suited to those for whom polio does not conclude but is a permanent present. The polio memoir (again, aimed as often toward the able-bodied as toward the polio-impaired reader) takes its reader into, through, and beyond the polio experience, while the polio newsletter productively and necessarily dwells within, building a new textual environment for its "new world of people," themselves in the process of developing a new polio reality.

In thinking about these earlier polio-affected communities as inaugurators of the modern disability rights movement, it is helpful to consider what modern critical studies of this issue have helped us to learn about such community formation. Specifically the findings of scholars of deafness as a bodily particularity and especially of Deaf culture as a proud and politically progressive "linguistic minority" bear productively on the phenomenon of rehabilitation culture and discourse that flourished mid-century at polio clinics and centers around the US. This cultural identity coincides with or may in some ways conflict with biological membership in a hearing family. Harlan Lane observes that Deaf culture is much less interested to mainstream or integrate "its own" children (i.e., deaf children from hearing or deaf families of school age); they argue that deaf teachers are best equipped to instruct such children in signing, reading, and writing and that these children's self-esteem and personal and social integration will come primarily from associating with the Deaf community. As Lane notes, "[o]rganizations espousing each construction of deafness [i.e., deafness as impairment and Deafness as cultural identity] compete to 'own' the children and define their needs."[4] Also Lennard J. Davis elaborates upon the concept of Deaf persons as a nation within a nation (in this case, the United States), drawing upon writers as diverse as Benedict Anderson and Josef Stalin to explore the idea of Deaf nationalism. In 1913, Stalin defined a nationality as having "(1) a common language; (2) a stable community; (3) a territory; (4) economic cohesion; (5) a collective psychology and character."[5] Most pertinent to this study, "Anderson thinks of nation as a manifestation of print culture. . . . [I]t was readers 'connected through print, [who] formed, in their secular, particular, visible invisibility the embryo for the nationally imagined community.'"[6]

While Davis reads Deaf culture according to these theories, they are equally helpful to understanding Williams and Laurie's "new world of people," the permanently polio-affected in postwar America, as is the ethnofamilial model of bodily particularity enacted by Deaf culture and theorized by Lane. Mid-century residents of polio rehabilitation centers did not meet Stalin's criterion of a "stable community," coming to these centers with the express purpose of leaving them rapidly and permanently behind. Yet many came as exiles from forward-moving, able-bodied America (what Davis calls "the United States of Ability")[7] and found life-sustaining collective and individual identities therein. For those who were never able to leave behind their status as physically impaired, their membership in these disability communities defined and oriented them throughout their lives; while they may have left the physical setting of the rehab centers themselves (their shared "territory," in Stalin's terms), they remained citizens of this invisible nation through the mobilizing force of its print culture.

Similar to the sign language that distinguishes and unites its Deaf practitioners, polio language will be read in this chapter as the particular ways in which those recovering from polio spoke to each other in a textual canon that only they were meant to read, only they were meant to understand. While it was not a language as specialized as ASL, it is characterized by a vocabulary whose terms would have mystified the non-polio-initiated, while its style was a product of the rehabilitation experience (its frustrations, absurdities, and occasions for dark humor) and the residents themselves, whose age and class demographics will be considered below. It is true that their "interpretive community" (Stanley Fish's term) included not only rehab center residents but their doctors, therapists, visiting family members, local and national politicians, and the advertisers who sometimes occupied the pages of even in-house newsletters (in addition to at least one polio-related national magazine, *Accent on Living*); I will argue, however, that the print culture of polio nationhood was most revolutionary, and most therapeutic, when it addressed itself specifically to the polio-affected community. Its adult and juvenile members recognized in such writing their shared, permanent membership in an exclusive, even privileged society, empowering themselves through such membership even as they returned, as crutch-walkers, wheelchair-rollers, and iron-lung-breathers, to the outside world.

Earliest Issues

In many ways the *Polio Chronicle* reflected the character of the stately, benevolent patrician who presided not only over its board of trustees but, a few years after the newsletter's inception, the nation as a whole.[8] Roosevelt was only governor of New York when the *Chronicle* kicked off

VOL. 2 *April*, 1933 NO. 9

The Polio Chronicle

Recording the Crusade Against Poliomyelitis (Infantile Paralysis)

International News Photo

ROOSEVELT TAKES OATH AS 32ND PRESIDENT

President Franklin D. Roosevelt takes the oath of office as 32nd President of the United States. Chief Justice Charles E. Hughes is shown administering the oath as ex-President Herbert Hoover (right) looks on.

Official Organ of the POLIO CRUSADERS, a national movement against Infantile Paralysis. Published monthly by the NATIONAL PATIENTS' COMMITTEE, a voluntary organization of persons who are victims of Infantile Paralysis, with headquarters at the GEORGIA WARM SPRINGS FOUNDATION, Warm Springs, Georgia.

Subscription Price, $1.00 a Year.

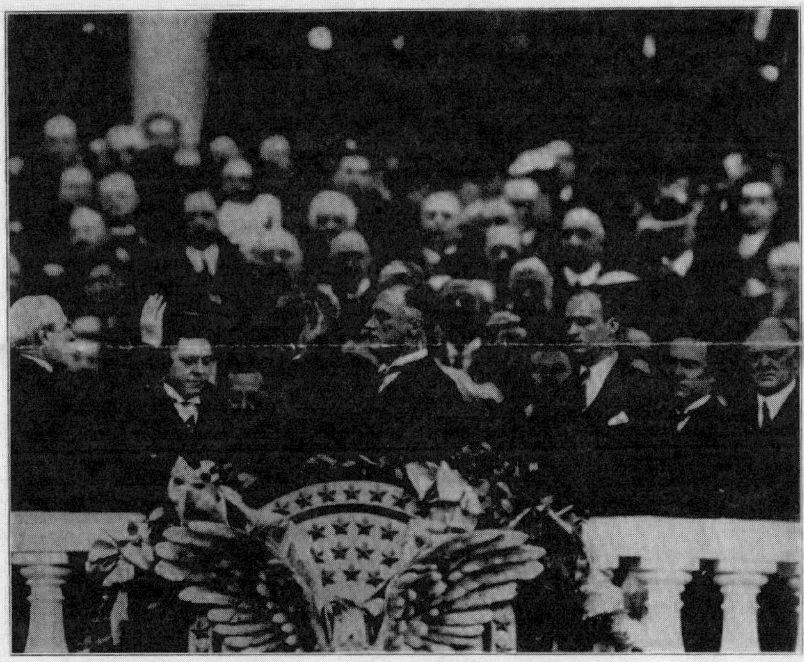

Figure 1. *The Polio Chronicle,* April 1933. Courtesy of Roosevelt Warm Springs Institute for Rehabilitation, Warm Springs, Georgia.

in 1931; his ascent to the presidency was celebrated in its pages by both Democrats and Republicans at Warm Springs (December 1932; see also figure 1), whose party affiliations took a backseat to their loyalties to the Foundation's founding father.[9] In these early days, especially before he became president, Roosevelt made frequent visits to Warm Springs, pervading its sultry, backwoods atmosphere with an air of refinement and providing the occasion to spruce up, cheer up, and keep up a class act in every particular. Considering the ways Roosevelt sought to disguise or deny his polio disability throughout his life, Davis argues that "Since the disabled are a kind of minority group within the nation, it would hardly do for the President to be a representative of that minority group."[10] Although his argument is true in many ways, it is the case that Roosevelt was known and loved by his fellow-polio survivors as one of their own. His identity as "a polio" and his frequent presence at Warm Springs had a gentrifying effect not only on those lucky enough to be residents at Warm Springs but on those affected by polio and the otherwise-physically impaired across the nation. As far as concerned this minority group itself, Roosevelt indeed represented them figuratively and literally; he was president not only of the able-bodied United States but founding father of an ever-grateful polio nation.

Likely, the dignified styling of this early serial reflected the upper-class status of many of the Foundation's first residents as well. In the early '30s, the organization that would become the March of Dimes was little more than a twinkle in Roosevelt's eye, and the only ones able to afford an extended, rehabilitative stay at this former resort—especially in the heart of the Depression—were likely to be as wealthy and as socially connected as was Roosevelt himself. Photos in the *Chronicle* of polio achievers who returned from Warm Springs to positions of power featured men in suits and ties, women with styled hair and stylish hats. The masthead was set in gothic type, suggesting a fraternity with *The New York Times*; an early contributor of medically detailed articles was John Ruhrah, M.D., who was himself a "Foundation member" (i.e., patient) and a source of copious technical information. The residents' elite status was reinforced by the stark racial stratification of the Foundation: "colored" and "negro" persons served the food and entertained on numerous occasions, according to the *Chronicle*'s coverage of social events, and even the most adversely affected Warm Springs resident could feel himself superior to these othered classes. Small wonder then that the *Chronicle*'s editorial staff, and the larger group of residents who did much of the programming at Warm Springs, named themselves the "National

Patients' Committee": not only were they representative of, and singularly privileged among, the thousands recovering from polio in America at that time; they also bore the imprimatur of the nation's leader at a moment when polio was little less than the national disease.

In a striking editorial in the April 1933 issue, the editors fend off criticism that "the CHRONICLE is too dry, that it lacks the proportion of humorous and light material to make it interesting to all." Yet they agree to include more material on "the humorous side of polio," significantly, for its therapeutic effects: "Interesting events are part of the Crusade, for they show how we here compensate for losses of athletics, etc. The funny incidents and accidents are a part of our attitude toward polio." Their concession is a page containing cartoons (featuring "Polio Pete"), reviews of the week's entertainment, and lists of visitors entitled "Bubbles from the Spring." The editors even try a limerick or two in what seemed to be a recurring "Paralyzing Poetry!" feature. Meanwhile, they are resolute in their refusal to include items of a gossipy nature: "The fact that Bill Jones went to Columbus with Mary Smith is not an important step in this Crusade" and would likely draw disdain from "[t]he host of doctors, nurses, and physiotherapists who make up a large part of our circulation."

Yet it is necessary to question the idea that publishing personal tidbits about the residents' personal lives and romantic escapades would play no part in the anti-polio crusade. "Bill and Mary's" elopement would surely have terrific curative effect for the couple themselves, while reporting upon it would only multiply the payoff: not only are the little doings of seemingly unimportant rehab center residents now seen to be of vital significance, but the readership itself makes a vicarious escape with this happy couple and may more seriously contemplate their own prospects for romantic fulfillment because of it. Perhaps most important (or at least most likely), Bill and Mary become household names to the larger community, who await their return, and the occasion to harass them, with raucous anticipation. Both individual identities and communal connections are formed through disseminating gossip in such a publication; the *Chronicle* refused to admit this possibility, but its several successors took up this particular campaign in the Crusade with zeal.

THE LIGHTER TOUCH

Warm Springs' second installation, *The Crutch*, had by the late 1930s supplanted the *Chronicle* and took itself far less seriously. The mast was in simple font and the plain type loosely spaced. Headlines, paragraph breaks, and cut-lines of various widths broke up verbal monotony; football scores and a children's column are front-page features of the November 15, 1937 issue (see figure 2). In fact children played almost no role in the sophisticated pages of the *Chronicle*; as the Warm Springs newsletter moves through its later permutations, they will be an ever-more central feature, and the adults will come off more and more youthfully, even childishly on occasion, making this community seem even more unified and solidified in its exuberant outlook, its shared tastes in news and entertainment.

This downshift in editorial styling coincides with the physical transformations undergone by the Foundation itself. In 1933, the stately but declining Meriwether Inn, which had been a Warm Springs spa/resort since the nineteenth century, was taken down and Georgia Hall (still on the grounds today) erected in its place. Interestingly, the Inn had been a site of tension during the Foundation's earliest days, when its able-bodied clientele looked with horror upon, then fled in disgust with, the encroaching population of polio rehabilitators who adapted its country club atmosphere to its own needs.[11] If the original polio-affected residents of Warm Springs were in fact an equally classy bunch whose elegant newsletter reflected the refined setting they were pleased to preserve, the collegiate air of the succeeding *Crutch* conveys the sense that Warm Springs itself had transformed into an environment akin to a well-run college—more state-sponsored than Ivy League—by the late '30s as well. Marc Shell notes that "most communal institutions for polios were partly rehabilitative and partly academic and social." Shell quotes polio memoirist Lorraine Beim, who describes her "acceptance letter" to Warm Springs, received the same year she received an acceptance letter to Wheaton College. Beim writes, "Warm Springs . . . is in many ways like a college.'"[12]

Considering the issue of social class as it may be traced in the styling of these newsletters, it is helpful to return to Davis who argues persuasively for the connection between disability and class: "disability causes poverty, and . . . poverty likewise causes disability,"[13] due to the hazardous nature of low-level work and lack of access to medical care for those in the lower classes. It is also the case that disability oftentimes impoverishes even middle-class and wealthy persons, due to the toll taken on personal finances to sustain an adequate post-impairment lifestyle. This funding issue is exactly what caused Williams and Laurie to approach the federal government in 1961; significantly, however, in the

THE CRUTCH

VOL. 1. NO. 3 MONDAY, NOV. 15, 1937 A WEEKLY PUBLICATION

THE MOVIE WEEK
By Paul Rogers

MONDAY: THE SINGING MARINE. Warner Bros. best musical of the season, starring their favorite crooner, Dick Powell. In addition to Powell, who is above the average in this picture, the music is pleasing, the comedy is comic (Hugh Herbert, Jane Darwell, and Allen Jenkins). Also a newcomer (Doris Weston) who sings naturally and is easy on the eyes. She arrived via Major Bowes' hour. Also on this bill, Charlie McCarthy on his second visit to Cumerford.

THURSDAY: CAPTAINS COURAGEOUS. Kipling's favorite adventure story lives again, with a cast of stars. Freddy Bartholomew, Spencer Tracy, Lionel Barrymore, Melvyn Douglas. This outstanding MGM poduction makes a bid for a place among the immortals.

SATURDAY MATINEE: NEW FACES OF 1937. For the Joe Penner, Milton Berle, Parkyakarkus fans. An RKO musical comedy.

SATURDAY EVENING: Carole Lombard and Fred MacMurray in HANDS ACROSS THE TABLE, being a second showing of this very amusing Paramount farce-comedy.

CHILDREN'S NEWS
By Janice Howe

HOW I GOT MY DOG

One rainy evening we were sitting around the fireplace. We heard a tiny whimpering outside the door. We opened the door and there sat a little puppy dog all wet, curled up and full of mud.

We took him inside and gave him a warm bath and some milk to drink. After that I put him on a warm rug to sleep. His color was white with black pots all over him. He had a black spot over his right eye. So I named his "Blackeye". He was such a cute little pup that we did not have the heart to send him away. I was very much afraid somebody would take him away from me but nobody wanted him, and I could keep him.

So this is how I got my dog, "Blackeye".

—ROBERT ROSENBAUM.

Foundation To Attend Football Game
By Robert E. Shermer

Mr. Fred Botts, Registrar, this morning informed THE CRUTCH that arrangements are being completed with Mr. L. W. McPherson, of Columbus, Ga., whereby patients and staff members of the Foundation will be admitted to the football game between The Alabama Polytechnic Institute (Auburn) and The University of Georgia, next Saturday, as complimentary guests of the Georgia-Auburn Football Association.

Every comfort and consideration for the Foundation family is being arranged, with a motorcycle escort meeting the motorcade on Hamilton Road, on the outskirts of Columbus, and from the stadium.

Weather permitting, a very large crowd is anticipated, as this is doubtless one of the finest games to be played anywhere in stadia this Fall throughout the South.

Foundationites have attended this great fiesta en masse in previous years and have enjoyed themselves to the very utmost. This year should prove no exception.

Will all persons planning to attend please signify their intentions by contracting either the Registrar or THE CRUTCH at once so that the exact number of automobiles can be adequately provided? Further details will be announced Monday and Tuesday in the Dining Hall. Likewise announcements will appear on the Bulletin Board in Georgia Hall.

In Memoriam
HAROLD BURT
1906-1937

It is with infinite sadness that we record the passing of Harold Burt, of Jamestown, New York, whose death came Wednesday evening after a six-day struggle against pneumonia. To his mother, Mrs. F. C. Burt, we extend our sincerest sympathy.

Light 'Iron Lung' Invented To Aid Victims of Polio

A new lightweight respirator, developed by Dennis Scanlon, Akron, Ohio, inventor, may relieve Frederick B. Snite, Jr., 27-year-old infantile paralysis victim, from the cumbersome "iron lung" which has been his home for 19 months, it was learned today.

Scanlon telephoned the Snite residence in Miami from Akron last night and gave a detailed description of the "lung." Frederick B. Snite, Sr., father of young Fred, was not home when Scanlon called, but said he understood the respirator would be tested here early next week.

Descriptions of the new "lung" indicate it is similar to a Swedish chest respirator that was tried unsuccessfully here recently, he said. "Neither Fred nor I can get excited over it until it has been tried out, because we receive calls and letters about things like that every day."

At present young Snite is encased in a Drinker respirator which covers his entire body, only his head protruding. It has been his home since he was stricken with the paralysis in China 19 months ago. Scanlon's respirator is designed to give young Snite free use of his arms and legs.

Football Scores

(Friday night, Nov. 12)

Mercer 20	Tampa 0
Miami (Fla.) 21	Catholic U. 0
Wake Forest 24	Wofford 0
Coe 7	Grinnell 0
B'ham-Sou. 38	Spring Hill 0
R. I. State 13	Providence 0
Kansas Wesleyan 19	Baker 6

GEORGIA
VS.
AUBURN
NOVEMBER 20, 1937
COLUMBUS, GEORGIA
ON TO COLUMBUS NOV. 20TH!

Figure 2. The Crutch, November 15, 1937. Courtesy of Roosevelt Warm Springs Institute for Rehabilitation, Warm Springs Georgia.

1940s and 1950s when Warm Springs was in its polio heyday, the nationwide polio community's "economic cohesion" (returning once more to Stalin's terminology) came from the well-run and generously supportive March of Dimes, allowing even those profoundly affected the necessary medical care and living standards, enabling Warm Springs and centers like it around the country to assume an air much less of boot camp (or internment camp) than of summer camp. Shell's report of the "acceptance letter" to Warm Springs indicates that such rehabilitation centers were in their own way elite clubs that selected members based on specific criteria—race, unfortunately, remaining a primary one and the limited number of spaces being another. Beyond that, one's impairment status seemed to be the main determinant; one senses from newsletters of this period that Warm Springs (and other rehab centers such as Rancho Los Amigos in Hondo, California) served the white middle and working classes and that this fundamental divide (between, in another register, bourgeoisie and proletariat) closed easily in the all-against-polio setting.[14]

Not only were regional football contests a more and more pressing concern in the *Crutch*; the Warm Springs "campus" itself provided its "students" with the spectrum of programming commonly associated with colleges as institutions of character formation: clubs, teams, contests, trips, entertainments, and service opportunities galore—indeed, everything but actual classes—are reported upon frequently in the pages of the *Crutch*. Interestingly, "course work" in this context would have been the rehab sessions each patient subjected himself to—the stretching, exercise, swimming, and difficult, endless practice that were in fact rarely mentioned in this publication. Its heavy coverage of leisure activities—a debate club, nightly films, a Beautiful Eyes contest, prizes on Washington's Birthday for "most original headdress"—depict Warm Springs residents during this period as overgrown kids playing hooky, which for necessary, therapeutic reasons they in fact were. In an early issue, the editors christened the *Crutch* "a nonofficial publication,"[15] seeming to thumb their noses at the trenchant officialism of the preceding *Chronicle* and to invite readers to enjoy as best they could a sanctioned break from official roles.

To be sure, the *Crutch* continued to scatter among its lighter fare the informative, more serious articles that were a central feature of the *Chronicle*. One news item described the latest in respirator technology—offered first, not surprisingly, to Frederick Snite, Jr., likely the wealthiest respiratory polio survivor in U.S. history[16]—while another piece in the same issue gave a historical overview of rehabilitation services since the nineteenth century.[17] What looks at first like a "Dear Abby" column in fact treats a vital political issue—"shall polios marry?"—and includes a range of responses; unfortunately, even Foundation residents interviewed for the piece feel that "mixed" marriages—a "polio" and an "A.B." (able body)—were likely to fail.[18] Like its predecessor the *Chronicle*, the *Crutch* maintained a connection to the larger world by including letters each week (mostly in praise of the *Crutch*) from prominent subscribers—among them Roosevelt and Snite—and reporting heavily on visitors' comings and goings. In one strangely slanted item from the "Personals" column that listed these many arrivals from the outside, even the death of a resident is reframed in terms of a visit from his sister, "called to the Foundation Wednesday" to evidently collect the dead man's body.[19] Clearly an element of denial is at work in the wording of this entry, though other questions remain open: was this cultivated connection to the able-bodied world the more therapeutic method for such a publication to employ, or would the intense inward focus of its successor, the *Wheelchair Review*, prove the more restorative textual approach?

If these personals were in fact fairly public in their orientation after all, another recurring installment, "Scene and Heard Here and There," delves into the gossip surrounding the residents themselves that the editors of the *Chronicle* decried. The column's title tells all: this extensive collection of glimpses and over-hearings, gathered by two reporters whose informant network must have been extensive, mimics the scintillating buzz of society columns and celebrity tabloids. The reporters and their informants clamored like paparazzi for the latest tip, and those lucky enough to be featured from one issue to the next may have bristled at the intrusion but enjoyed the adulation as well. That *every* resident got to be the celebrity at some point in these writings breaks down the traditional dichotomy between sought-after star and obscure, anonymous public. At Warm Springs, and likely since their first days with polio, residents' basic rights to privacy barely existed; being featured in an admiring write-up might have been a welcome change from their typical role as specimen for probing physicians and therapists. In the gossip columns, everyone felt himself the fascinating center of attention on a regular basis, an effective antidote to the anxieties of being forgotten and ignored upon return to the able-bodied world. And the marked triviality of these items—one resident did not like last night's movie; doesn't another one have a pretty smile?—would tend to boost the ego even more: every little thing one was and did was of interest to this close-knit community, yet one had to be or do nothing very special at all to be a topic of such gratifying mention.

Special attention surrounded gossip of a romantic nature, which in turn raised the question of whether these published pryings had in fact overstepped their bounds, had violated rights to private courtship and sexual activity taken for granted in the able-bodied world. While what a male and female patient "sitting on the floor of the bus" were "seen and heard" doing remains unclear, the reference is more pointed, and both more juvenile and more suggestive, in a later item: "No doubt most of you don't know what the uproar was last Sunday evening at the push-boys' table—Well it's like this: [name]'s lips were red, and believe me, he hadn't been eating strawberries."[20] Pushboys were able-bodied staff members who pushed patients in wheelchairs around the Foundation; on occasion they married the female residents, yet the "uproar" following this tryst involving a staff member does not indicate any such serious attachment. From these polio publications, one learns that sex between residents and between staffers and residents was a fairly frequent occurrence at Warm Springs; in one issue of the *Wheelchair Review*, one patient suggests "more bushes and fewer lights" (bushes being the classic site for romantic assignations) when asked about more recreational activities.[21] That some of this sexual activity exploited the women involved is a possibility, and this possibility, joked away in the item quoted above, complicates the issue of staff ethics of conduct, as well as the newsletter's own journalistic responsibilities or breach thereof.

Indeed the *Wheelchair Review* indulged even more frequently and more variously than did the *Crutch* in speculating on residents' romantic and sexual goings-on; much of the writing involved such tattling on who was seen with whom, who was crying over whom, who (or what) was driving whom crazy. Most of the ribbing was good-natured, though not without its edge: one resident, a former medical student, is reported to suffer from "acute dementia praecox with schizophrenic tendencies," and to have been visited by "the Foundation's recently acquired psychologist."[22] However, the comment derails into a gag—a list of the eccentric activities engaged in by the patient, including cutting out paper dolls—yet a somewhat cruel one, inviting laughter at the patient's expense just as it touches on the sore point of his regrettably preempted medical career. In a "pet peeves" column patients harass each others' baseball teams, criticize obnoxious behavior, and name fellow-residents specifically among their peeves. The newly arrived were shielded from the merciless kidding, as items on "newcomers" had a much more neutral, welcoming tone than items referred to as "news"—gossip and teasing by and about Warm Springs veterans. Yet even "Crutch Tips and Brace Points," offered in the same issue, both attempts to con the greenhorns with comic misinformation and criticizes the uncaring staff: "For you men to get a push boy, be sure to wear a wig and skirt, act helpless and push your chair in front of you. . . . Friday is the only day you can duck your therapist—the beauty shop is most accommodating and likes the trade. . . . If you really want service, get a television set in your room."[23]

Even more pointed is a satiric essay entitled "Pushboys, Arise!," which calls for these neglectful attendants to get off their "divans" and do some actual attending. Mid-essay, the author gently prods, "It's hard to preach the Golden Rule to a group of lads who don't fully realize how much they mean to us. But it becomes annoying every so often to be obliged to cater to the whims of the preoccupied pushboy. Just because we can't very well exact retribution is no reason to take advantage of us, boys."[24] Exploitation by an indifferent staff, speculated upon above in my discussion of one pushboy's "red lips," and the resultant disgruntlement of the patients depending on them seems to have been widespread at this point and may account in part for the rougher tone of these pages.

Perhaps the most striking theme specific to the *Review* is the residents' bracing focus (pun intended) on their bodies and physical situations. No longer are the reporters and interviewees inclined to silence on the glaring issue of their reason for being at Warm Springs; the increased interest in residents' love lives is part of this new comfort with the body and its travails, as are their pet peeves related to inattendant pushboys, unappetizing therapeutic diets, "my little ol' iron corset," and "P.T.'s who lie awake nights dreaming of new exercises for my already tired muscles."[25] "Glute" jokes (regarding weak gluteus muscles) are a staple, and an accomplished author in residence claims that he would "trade his Ph.D. for an A.B. [able body] any day!"[26] The "Eaters Club" offered its members the chance to maintain contacts among residents in a post-rehab context. Residents and alumni were invited to mail in for a "club card": "[b]y presenting this card to any other member, one is entitled to a free meal."[27] The club created a members' directory, an early attempt to use texts—the directory, the club card—to maintain vital support networks as polio survivors reintegrated into the "A.B." world. This would be the primary aim of polio "lifestyle" magazines published in the post-polio context, like the *Toomey j. Gazette* (references to which opened this chapter) and the "twelve-page magazine" published by Polio Parents, Inc. a self-help group in Swarthmore, Pennsylvania, for polio survivors and their families.[28]

In the *Review* B. Sinclair's cheeky column (actually, an entire page) "For Skirts Only," provides women advice not only on gadgets like reaching tools and lap boards helpful to both sexes (a beat covered thoroughly by *Accent on Living* and the *Gazette* as well) but beauty tips that acknowledge women's special challenge of maintaining marriageable femininity despite their new limitations. Sinclair advises on the most wearable fashions for wheelchairs (separates and wrap-around skirts), attractive enough to "draw the observer's interest away from the disability"; feminine touches any woman might add—a rope of pearls converted into a choker, the latest color for fall ("rhubarb"), and "a gold sequin at the outer tip of each eyebrow for the evening"[29]—connected female readers to their able-bodied counterparts by presenting them with "normal" feminine options, especially from the waist up. While the present-day able-bodied feminist perspective frowns upon such "girl talk," the disability-studies feminist standpoint includes serious inquiry into the difficulty impaired women have had, especially in the modern era, finding sex and marriage partners.[30] Mairian Corker and Sally French define the role of discourse in disability studies in explicitly feminist terms.[31] The discourse I attempt to claim here is the body of rehabilitation writing as a whole, as well as women-focused columns such as Sinclair's.

In a long, descriptive piece in the *Review* called "Now You Know," Bill Tyndale provides a complete list of the splints, slings, crutches, braces, and other assistive devices conceived and fabricated by the Warm Springs brace shop, praising the inventiveness, specificity, and effectiveness of each piece developed. The list itself indicates the vast spectrum of requirements supported by these many devices; Tyndale distinguishes between the able-bodied view of "'men from mars' get-ups" that cause a "reserved but polite shudder," and the polio survivor's understanding that these devices were not confining but liberating, not gruesome but "beautiful in the respect of being real art produced by the hands and ingenuity of master craftsman [*sic*]."[32] Tyndale implicitly advises his readership to consider their assistive devices as the one-of-a-kind folk (or "outsider") art objects that they in fact were, to wear them proudly but also subversively, counter-culturally, when they returned to the able-bodied sphere, as piercings and tattoos are worn as a statement of political dissidence today.

The *Review*'s remarkable cover art—a new line drawing by a resident artist for each issue—augments this focus on the body, its impairment and rehabilitation. Tyndale, Rozell Mink, and Janet Land provided humorous or inspiring sketches in the early 1950s; Jack Lightfoot's more sophisticated, densely shaded works from 1956 were even darker in their humor—a therapist exercising a patient with a sadistic grin, another patient with a postop leg stitched on backwards—and coincided with the *Review*'s adoption of a heavier-handed style reminiscent of the over-serious *Chronicle*. Later issues of the *Review* include a full page for table of contents, a lengthy staff listing, and subscription rates, details too elaborate for what was still just a fifteen-page packet. At this point, the newsletter also returned to longer, even full-page articles instead of the breezy, digestible items of the early 1950s. The single-panel gags featuring Polio Pete in the *Chronicle* of the '30s transformed into a full-length strip, "The Adventures of Polio Man," in late 1956. While production style remained grassroots, the over-serious attempt to copy commercial magazine format took the publication in the wrong direction, bogging it down, stilting its ad hoc, fast-paced flow. By contrast, earlier drawings by Tyndale, Mink, and Land moved airily across the page: Mink penned a comical four-panel "New Patients Views Of Warm Springs" (May 14, 1955; see figure 3), each containing a view of the ceiling—light fixtures, the roof of the brace shop, etc.—as seen from a stretcher. Tyndale decorated the cover of the President's Day 1952 issue with George Washington, ax raised—not cutting down a cherry tree, but gleefully hacking his wheelchair (see figure 4). Land's cover for the March 12, 1955 issue (selected for the cover of this book as well) connotes energy and freedom—a charming boy whizzing downhill in his wheelchair, aided by his lofty kite and a bracing gust from Mr. Wind.

Perusing the staff listings of various issues across the decades reveals the rapidly revolving door that put new editors, reporters, and artists in charge almost from one week to the next. A flexible, minimalist publication style seems to have served best; cumbersome formatting worked against the requirements of the genre and took up space better devoted to maintaining those vital communication lines. The very existence of these publications, their reliable appearance on a weekly or daily basis, was continuity enough, and overproduction was simply a distraction as it was introduced and distracting yet again when it was removed or redesigned in the following issue. The lively, slapdash cover art and content pages of the early-fifties *Wheelchair Review*s may be seen to represent the pinnacle of the form at Warm Springs. The disgruntled voices, dark

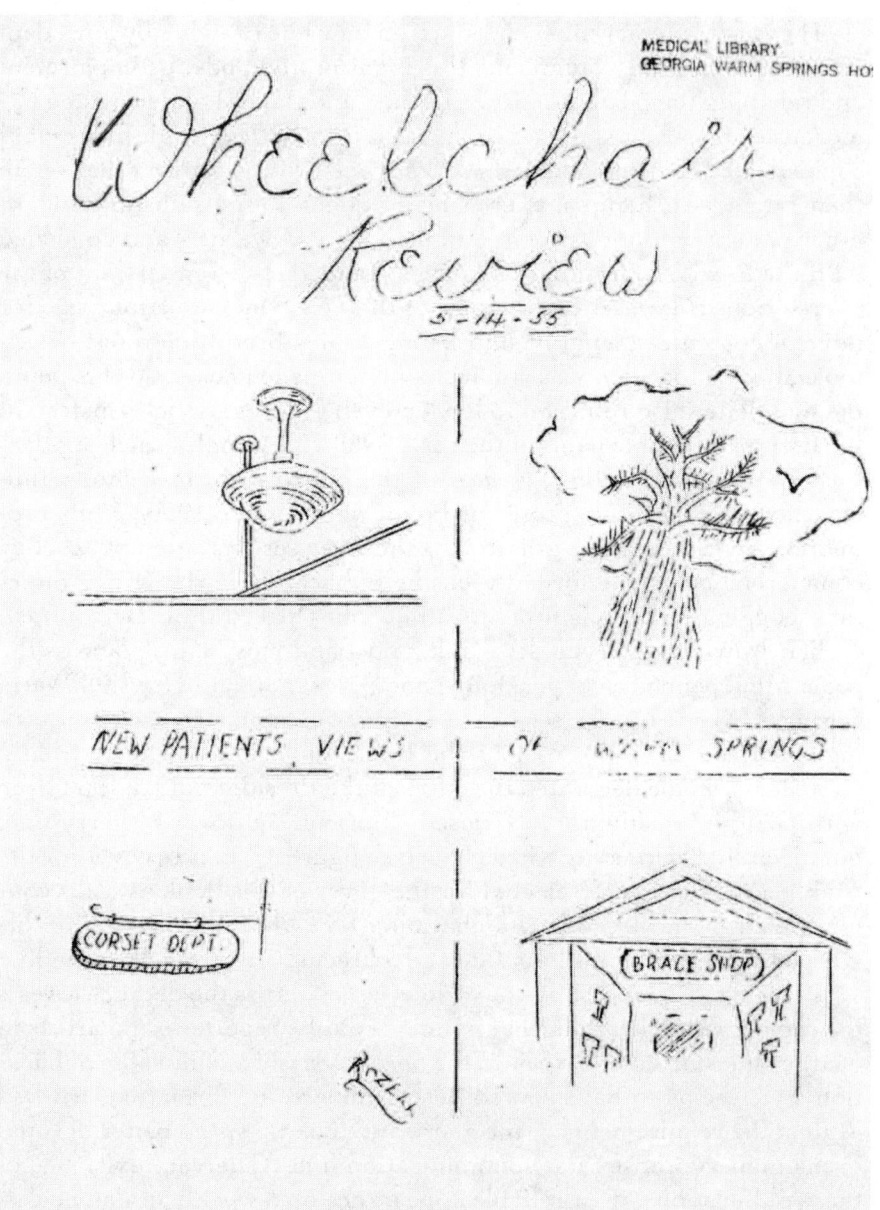

Figure 3. Rozell Mink, artist. *The Wheelchair Review,* May 14, 1955. Courtesy of Roosevelt Warm Springs Institute for Rehabilitation, Warm Springs Georgia.

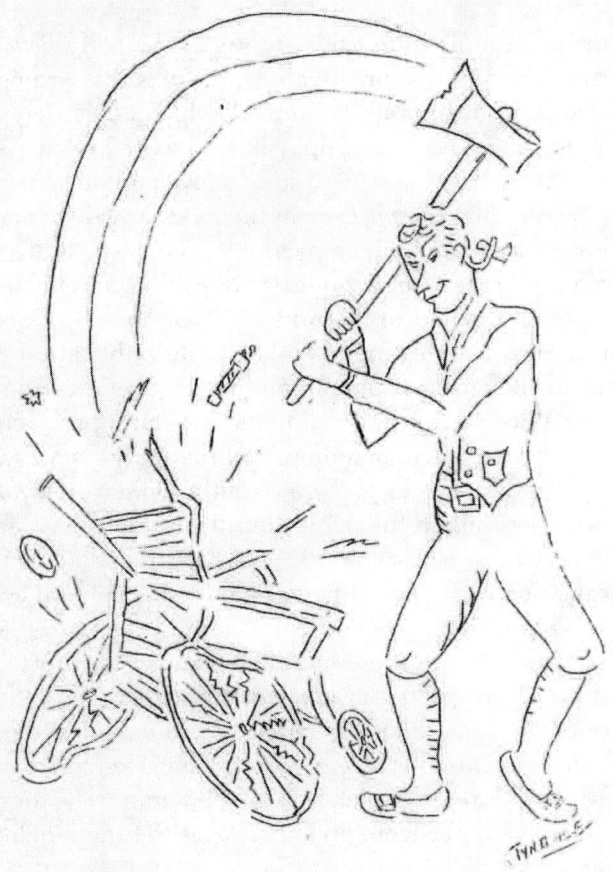

Figure 4. Bill Tyndale, artist. *The Wheelchair Review,* February 23, 1952. Courtesy of Roosevelt Warm Springs Institute for Rehabilitation, Warm Springs Georgia.

humor, and body-consciousness are most realistic and most therapeutic, suggesting in every particular lightheartedness, movement, and freedom.[33]

The Therapeutic Routine

One factor in the more expensive styling of the early *Polio Chronicle* (in addition to numerous ads for "invalid" products that provided an actual budget) was its monthly publication schedule, a leisurely timetable allowing reporters to do careful, sophisticated work and allowing more resources overall to be devoted to just a few annual issues. The many weeks separating one *Chronicle* from the next, however, also meant that this newsletter was much less a part of the communal life and the individual recovery process than would be one of more regular appearance. The *Crutch* in fact began in the mid 1930s as the *Daily Crutch*, a single sheet, listing that day's events. While a daily publication might indeed serve as the ideal constant companion for the loneliest and most traumatized among Warm Springs's residents, the daily production schedule was evidently too hectic to maintain, and the *Daily Crutch* soon gave way to a weekly *Crutch*, which, given a slightly longer interval to regroup, was able to offer a much fuller product. Both the *Crutch* and the *Review* seemed to have been weekly publications until the late 1950s, when the *Review*'s transition to a bimonthly was part of the general leave-taking of polio occurring both at Warm Springs and in the nation as a whole at that point. In addition to providing the most constant form of emotional support, the daily newsletter is also most coincident with the day-in-day-out nature of the rehabilitation experience. Had a daily issuance even become tedious eventually, it only would have been in line with the endless repetition of stretches, exercises, and minutely incremental improvements in the move from polio paralysis to functionality undergone by the residents themselves.

Beyond the rehab setting, polio is a daily (sometimes even minute-by-minute) experience for those who continue dealing with its residual effects; those most severely affected physically or emotionally might have felt the loss of not only fellow-residents sharing goals but the weekly newsletters that themselves bound this community through language, art, and humor. Warm Springs was in fact only one rehabilitation center that created community through text in this way: Rancho Los Amigos's *Weakly Breather* and the Buffalo Polio Respiratory Center's *Gulper's Gazette* (a comic reference to an air-swallowing method that allowed some respirator users periods of unassisted breathing) are just two examples of cleverly titled publications that vitally served the respiratory polio population of their regions.[34] Of course another daily "newsletter" is one's local paper, and a striking text from the early 1980s, E. Clinton Belknap's *Nebraska and the Fight Against Polio, 1944–65*, anthologizes what seems to have been every reference to polio statewide in twenty-one years. This collection is an interesting hybrid of low production values (the paste-up format, lack of supporting "scholarship," local, in fact private, publication), official reporting from statewide papers, and enormous cultural significance. It is a singular textual example (to my knowledge, no citizen of any other state ever compiled such a document) made out of hundreds of smaller items, many of which featured standard, recurring themes (the latest hospitalizations, visits from polio dignitaries, obituaries).

This exhaustive collection indicates that mention of polio in local papers—in Nebraska and likely nationwide—was frequent enough to have been oppressive. Even as certain polio clinic newsletters, like the Charlottetown *Polio Post*,[35] filled their pages with escapist fare, able-bodied readers of Nebraska's local papers during these decades may have felt as if there was nowhere to run from the endless train of bad news related to polio. It is plausible that polio was its own beat for one or more reporters at these local papers, so constant was the contact with area hospitals and March of Dimes chapters, which provided continuing updates. Belknap's cramped arrangement of columns appropriately reconstructs the claustrophobia no doubt created by the barrage of polio notices. Yet this coverage provided "vital" information that kept communities united (even if united in anxiety and grief) and informed with respect to fellow-citizens, near neighbors, and even family members whose infectious polio status, or tragic polio demise, removed them from personal contact.

Significantly, once the patient-generated newsletter transcended its origins in the rehab/outpatient setting to enjoy a professional (even commercialized) existence as an inter/nationally circulated magazine, it reached out to a far wider audience as it simultaneously withdrew from frequent circulation. None of the polio-related magazines discovered in my search appeared more often than once a month; publisher-editor Raymond Cheever's *Accent on Living* (which began its career as *Polio Living*)[36] was in fact quarterly, while the *Gazette*'s schedule changed over the years, being sometimes monthly, sometimes seasonal, and for more than a decade annual. As essential a source as these publications continued to be, readers reconnected with this vital textual community and the news and information it provided only at lengthy intervals. *Accent*'s "Idea Exchange" invited readers to present dilemmas that fellow-readers ruled on in the following issue. The *Gazette* used its "Letters" column to perform a similar function. Note, however, that the lag time between a question or call for assistance and its appropriate response could be two to six months (depending upon whether answers were provided by readers in time for the next issue), stilting the dialogue. Could a question even be remembered, would a problem seem so urgent, so many months after it had been posed? While those vitally involved in the question at hand—submitting it themselves or simply sharing it silently, busily searching for answers or responding because disagreeing with suggestions already published—faced a frustrating wait for the discussion to play out, those less involved (not having the problem being discussed, for instance) would be less frustrated than bored by the slow pace. As necessary as were these serial publications to readerships interested to connect with others in their situation, the lines of communication were surely attenuated by cumbersome temporal logistics.

Inter/National Circulation

What these widely circulated magazines lacked in continuity, they made up for in geographical reach. Both *Accent* and the *Gazette* provided an international perspective, cultivating alliances with polio foundations and individual polio survivors from around the world. On two facing pages from the Spring 1959 issue, *Accent* invites its audience to write and subscribe to the *Polio-Revue L'Archipel* (of France) and includes an item with photographs on the sewing instruction received by a polio patient in India. Letters to the editors of the *Gazette* came from all over the world, and the editors were special friends of Jürgen Erbsleben, a young West German who at an early stage in his polio career took a history-making flight across Europe with nursing aides and the latest in respirator technology (Summer 1959). Proficiency in English seemed to be a prerequisite for communication with these magazines, surely a limitation that excluded many, though journals maintained their international correspondence with at least a core of non-native speakers. Surely the purpose behind this broad scope was to create and connect the largest possible "new world" of para- and quadriplegic polio survivors. As Davis describes sign language, and thus its citizenry of sign users, as "transnational,"[37] so these editors offered citizenship in this new world without regard for national identity, indicating that one's status as a polio survivor overrode traditional boundaries and enabled exchanges with friends from around the world that many Americans in their able-bodied yet isolationist mindset never sought to experience. In this respect, the bedbound polio survivor traveled more widely than many Americans ever would and understood more about the wider world as well. Earlier or later in their respective careers, both magazines also expanded horizons by writing and designing for a more generalized disabled/quadriplegic audience, with name changes for both (from *Polio Living* to *Accent on Living*, from *Toomey j. Gazette*—named for Toomey Pavilion, a respiratory polio clinic—to *Rehabilitation Gazette*) indicating this broader reach.

Both magazines reported frequently on the latest in assistive devices, although their differing emphases even within this area indicate their ultimately divergent styles, aims, and readerships. *Accent*'s address to a wide audience of polio survivors (the respirator-assisted as well as, perhaps especially, crutch-walkers and wheelchair-users) coincides with its more conservative style and content, while the comparatively more urgent situation of the *Gazette*'s more narrowly defined, specifically respiratory readership seems to have given rise to its more radical, outspoken editorial approach. Both magazines enjoyed the donation of a $1,400 portable respirator (from the same manufacturer in Boulder, Colorado) and both ran contests to determine which reader would be the lucky recipient. Certainly, this donation was part altruism and part calculated move on the part of the Thompson company—to inform these magazines' audiences as to the existence of its product; interestingly, the *Gazette* ran no actual advertisements but obliged the company with a favorable write-up of the donation and the contest, while *Accent* used ads in every issue to both inform readers as to the latest products and pay its bills. Assistive devices (hand-operated autos, therapeutic beds, wheelchair lifts) were the primary commodities sold in the pages of *Accent*, while even editorial matter like the "New Products and Services" column served an advertising function by directing readers to various stores where the equipment in question was sold.

The sometimes imperceptible blending of editorial and advertising content added to the comparative slickness of Cheever's publication, its sophisticated design and construction as well as its overtly commercial aims typical of mainstream magazines. I suggest that *Accent*'s more commercial aspect benefitted its audience as importantly as did its special-interest/grassroots elements: the magazine's emphasis on advertising delineated its readership as a powerful consumer market, ready to direct its still considerable income toward product suppliers and public facilities (and even gas stations; see below) willing to retool for its needs. The ads themselves were informative, providing potential buyers with a range of choices and perhaps the comforting sense that technology and industry were racing to meet their requirements. The *Gazette* provided such technical support without the use of advertising; they frequently described (and hand-drew) the latest in portable respirators and mouthsticks (with which respirator users could do everything from type to paint to scratch), which were the devices of greatest interest to their respiratory readership.

In addition to its use of advertising *Accent on Living* comes across as the more traditional publication in multiple respects. Stylistically, it offered few provocations, making use of traditional layouts and lettering; the *Gazette* often hand-wrote its "Bulletin Board" items, centering them on variously sized and shaped "scraps" and tacking them to a line-drawn bulletin board. Such inventive handwork made these regular "columns" into visually striking works of art; each page provided an eclectic mélange of font types, photography, hand-lettering, line-drawing, expressionistic angles, humor, and tragedy. *Accent* frequently discussed employing "the handicapped" and profitable lines of work for the newly impaired, though the wider range of income options available to *Accent*'s primarily less impaired readership made this a less urgent issue. By contrast, meaningful work and adequate income were almost obsessive themes for the *Gazette*, which reviewed and added to the most viable possibilities — mouth-painting greeting cards, selling magazines (and other items) over the phone, monitoring local TV stations (to report to advertisers whether their ads were shown as promised), and even graphology (handwriting analysis) — in every issue. The *Gazette* also ran several items on ham radio operating — a popular pastime in the 1950s that was appropriate for the fully paralyzed and an interesting means by which to connect respiratory ham operators with their able-bodied counterparts around the country.

Accent's regular features included advice to the lovelorn ("Dear Bonnie") and a spiritual column ("The Bible Says"). One progressively slanted article asked "Should the Handicapped Consider Marriage?" while the *Gazette* discussed "Sex and the Disabled."[38] That *Accent* was published by a wheelchair-using male editor says little if anything about the politics of the magazine he published, yet the *Gazette*'s being run by young women (three of whom were respirator users) suggests the *Gazette*'s origins in a groundbreaking collective of markedly atypical publishers. The contrasts enumerated here are not offered to subordinate the contribution made by *Accent* to that of the *Gazette*, nor to even suggest that *Accent* was politically conservative even though it was stylistically traditional. I wish instead to draw attention to the markedly different niches each occupied, the likely divergent audiences each served: traditional, middle-class, less polio-affected readers for *Accent*; more deeply involved respirator users for the *Gazette*, whose radically new physical circumstances perhaps overrode former class identifications and tastes in reading material, allowing all members of this new class to embrace the *Gazette*'s no-holds-barred style.

Despite its more traditional output, by the late 1960s *Accent* was publishing high-quality, civil rights-influenced articles advocating for access and acceptance for the physically impaired. Various issues directly address ableist prejudice;[39] William R. Scales's "Battle of the Bathroom"[40] treats a topic understandably enraging to wheelchair users with gracious good humor. Scales describes the pre-ADA nightmare of simply leaving home, knowing that bathrooms large enough to accommodate one's apparatus will be difficult if not impossible to find. The author chuckles over his having to use heavily trafficked facilities with the door open, getting stuck inside of an outhouse, and using women's bathrooms, which for mysterious reasons are often more spacious than men's. While he points out that he has become the devoted customer of one oil company whose gas station bathrooms are indeed large enough, he refrains from naming the company in question which might have had even more effect. Scales generously refuses to criticize the nonplussed able-bodieds who are surprised by and scowl upon his unorthodox bathroom visitations; his controlled approach to a topic others might attack with much more righteous indignation creates the optimal context for consciousness-raising among complacent ableists.

And let us observe the shifting significance of the "personal" focus that I found so therapeutic in the examples of the polio newsletters discussed above: where in those publications, the emphasis on an intensely networked polio community aided in the redevelopment of individual post-polio identities, here we observe that *Accent*'s early focus on the polio-affected (or otherwise impaired) *individual*—his employment options, his best bets with respect to mechanical assistance, his "personal problems"—represent the traditional (even politically conservative) approach to impairment and disability. The magazine's turn to the public aspects of the question—access, accountability, acceptance—is decidedly progressive in nature, and stands in sharp contrast to the "public relations" campaigns performed by early issues of the Warm Springs newsletters: these '30s-era appeals to the able-bodied sector prided themselves on maintained connections to it, pled to be remembered there; forty years later contributors to polio magazines lead the campaign to force awareness onto an indifferent mainstream and transfer the "problem" of disability from the individual to society.

As productive a piece of disability-rights journalism as Scales's article for *Accent* in fact is, it cannot help but pale a bit when compared to the more urgent agenda and exhilarated presentation of the *Gazette*. The earliest issues recall in detail the tone and content of the newsletters from Warm Springs, with continued strong interest in the littlest doings of its one-time residents. The "Toomey Alumni News" column refers to former residents' current health status and describes their post-polio lives. In a vein reminiscent of the most life-affirming numbers of Warm Springs's *Wheelchair Review*, the original aim of the *Gazette* is to share "fun" information with polio-affected respirator users from the Cleveland area and around the world.[41] The editors kid with one alumna who has not gotten around to reading the latest *Gazette* issue, and later that year editor Sue Williams chides readers for not only not reading their *Gazette*s but for failing to write back. In one issue a detailed lesson on frog-breathing (the gulping or air-swallowing method described above) is made "fun" by whimsical drawings of smiling frogs whose several speech balloons contain helpful hints from those who have mastered the difficult technique. Above I described the remarkably inventive "Bulletin Board" that was a recurring feature of the early issues; its design was eye-catching, its white-on-black lettering/illustration of the square, rectangular, even wedge-shaped and circular "notices" verged on the truly hip. One stylistic innovation that carried it through its middle years was the conversion from vertical, tabloid-style to a wide, short page that, when opened, presented a strikingly horizontal look. The editors explain that the magazine changed shape to rest better on the reading stands of iron lung users. In addition, of course, it perpetuates the horizontal worldview experienced by the majority of this respirator readership, reflecting lived experience in textual production as concretely as possible.

The Spring 1961 "Bulletin Board" exhorted its readers in the course of four separate items to "fill out CENSUS," "send in your CENSUS," and "drop us a card / We'll send you another" if you "LOST YOUR CENSUS"—the survey being one tool used by the editors to know and reach its citizenry (see figure 5). As if delegating responsibility at the meeting of a private club, the editors in another item ask their by-now

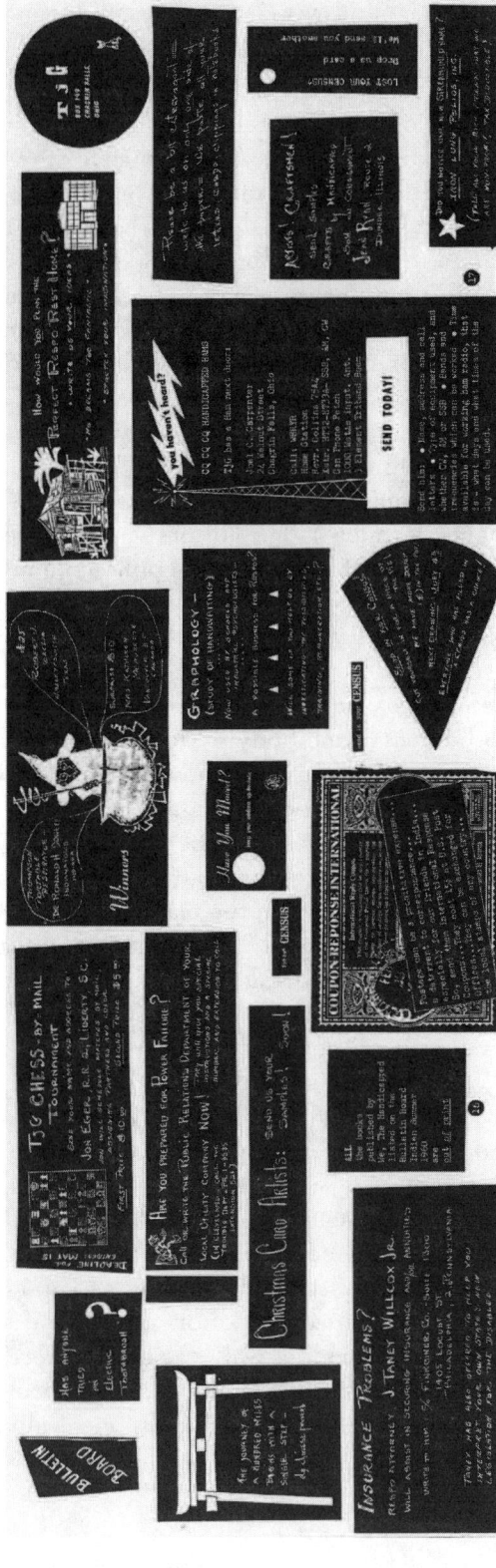

Figure 5. "Bulletin Board," Spring 1961. Courtesy of Post-Polio Health International.

international audience, "Will some of you help us by investigating the possibilities [of graphology as a career], training, remuneration, etc.?" Elsewhere, they solicit descriptions and drawings for the "perfect respo rest home,"[42] ask offhandedly "Did you notice our new . . . name?," and seek to connect "handicapped hams" (ham radio operators) to each other. Note the range in use value in these various announcements — from those constituting genuine information to those bearing purposely pointless chit-chat reminiscent of the most trivial detail-sharing of Warm Springs's later publications. Note also that each item requests and expects some sort of response from the reader — a reaching-out to other respirator users in the readership network or a writing-back to the editors themselves with information (about, for instance, graphology), ideas (about ideal rest homes), or more pointless chit-chat ("yes, I did notice your new name; it's nice"). The editors implicitly recognized that writing back was one thing this respiratory polio community did well, that interpersonal contact through reading, writing, and even radio operating had a new and essential function.

With a clever comment on the analogy between text and post-polio health, Sue Williams puns on the expression "level of involvement," which refers to both how (which body parts, to what degree) polio has affected a given person and, in this case, how actively involved with the newsletter a given reader may be. Williams jokes with her audience about the file cards kept on every subscriber: "To us," she informs, "the cards are not impersonal for we can pull out any one and rate it according to that person's involvement with the Gazette. How would the doctor-editors diagnoze [sic] your case?" Williams then outlines five levels of involvement, the most "fatal," being readerly disinterest: "(a) Against it — you're dead. Cause of death is suffocation." The healthiest scenario is "(e) Joins in by sending in a little news — you're not only healthy but you are still growing. We label you 'special people.'"[43] Another editor, Sally Russell, makes the case even more plainly: "We wish to bring to the readers stories and information that will be of real value to polios. . . . Friendship thru letter writing is a venture where polios have joined hands thru the pages of our magazine."[44] Finally, the "fourth wall" that so carefully limits the connection between any traditional magazine and its readership, lowered in each issue only as long as it takes to cull and (sometimes) reply to "Letters to the Editor," is rarely if ever visible in these earliest *Gazette*s. This dividing wall was barely there because (and I make this observation in the most complimentary respect possible), the *Gazette* was barely a magazine — text-based, yes, but as alive and personally present to its readers as otherwise possible in its looseness, informality, and proud non-professionalism.

And yet there is little of the triviality and silliness characterizing the "news" from Warm Springs to be found in this later publication. These respirator-using polio survivors' marked physical limitations distance them from their Warm Springs counterparts, whose impairments involving only the mid-section or various limbs seem by comparison a lighter load. The simplest activities described in the *Gazette*'s Alumni column, for instance, must be read also as major achievements; in fact these completely immobilized alumni are a remarkably mobile bunch, and the reportorial emphasis on their many activities—riding around in cars, visiting friends, touring Cleveland, watching an Indians ballgame—is as much "fun" to read about as it is startling and instructive. The able-bodied reader has the same reaction to the charming cartoons of Emmanuel Leplin, a Bay area composer of classical music and art editor for San Francisco's *Spokesman* (as in the spoke of a wheelchair wheel; see figure 6), yet another polio newsletter for and by polio survivors, one issue of which was reprinted in its entirety in the Spring 1960 *Gazette*. Leplin's drawings are spare but suggestive; his cartoon of a happily hooked-up respirator user—smiling at us with his portable chest shell respirator plugged into a wall—is arresting in its incongruity. It literally pictures the "adequate home care" called for in this panel that would put the smile on this polio survivor's face (see figure 7). One (the able-bodied one, that is) is taken further aback when the editors point out that all of Leplin's works are—no surprise after all—drawn by mouthstick. That Leplin makes more attractive, persuasive art with his mouth than most of us would make with both hands is another of those "fun" realizations that creates genuine awareness and understanding.

Epitomizing the humor, candor, and courage on regular display in these publications is Gini Laurie's *Gazette* editorial in the Summer 1959 issue, "Heads, you win!" With this marvelous pun (borrowed for my chapter's title), Laurie engages in a bit of potentially offensive slang only acceptable within this narrowly defined community. While not physically polio-affected herself, Laurie had lost three siblings to polio and was a long-time volunteer at the Toomey Pavilion clinic, a close friend of the "horizontal editors" who ran the *Gazette* as well, and a supporter of the local respiratory polio community in multiple ways. She was therefore as "in" within this community as a "vertical editor" could get, and her reference to them as "heads" indicates not only the closeness of her connection but the irreverent, forthright humor that seemed to have

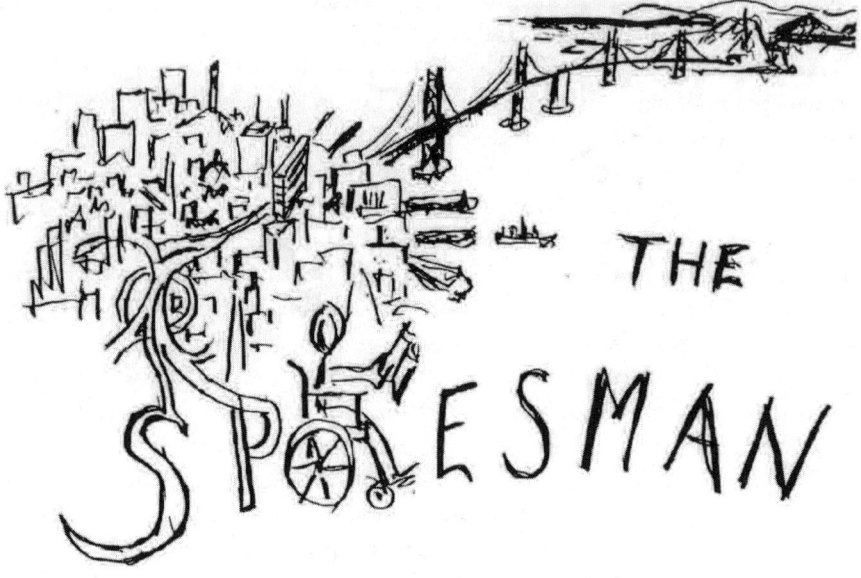

Figure 6. Emmanuel Leplin, artist. *The Spokesman* (rpt. *The Toomey j. Gazette,* Spring 1960). Courtesy of Rocky Leplin.

amused this group as a whole. Curiously, Laurie cannot fully escape her able-bodied status on this occasion, the blindspots that are its perennial hazards, as she addresses this column to able-bodieds like herself by referring to "my gentle, perceptive, fun-loving respiratory friends" and later (even more stridently) "these breathless characters" in the third person. As unfortunate as this angling of the address might be, Laurie nevertheless offers the profound reminder that, quoting Ecclesiastes, "wisdom is better than strength," that it is better to have one's head— even if that is all one has—than to be without it. If not like those respiratory polio survivors running around Cleveland with perfect disregard for their quadriplegic status, those, Laurie asserts, who simply "relax, enjoy life, and add depth to the lives of others" have "won" an important victory.

Shocking language coupled with taboo subject matter—specifically sex and death—in Dr. Duncan A. Holbert's article "Sex and the Disabled," drew a reaction of "horror and shock" from *Gazette* readers in 1967.[45] Yet Holbert calmly informs his readership that disabled people

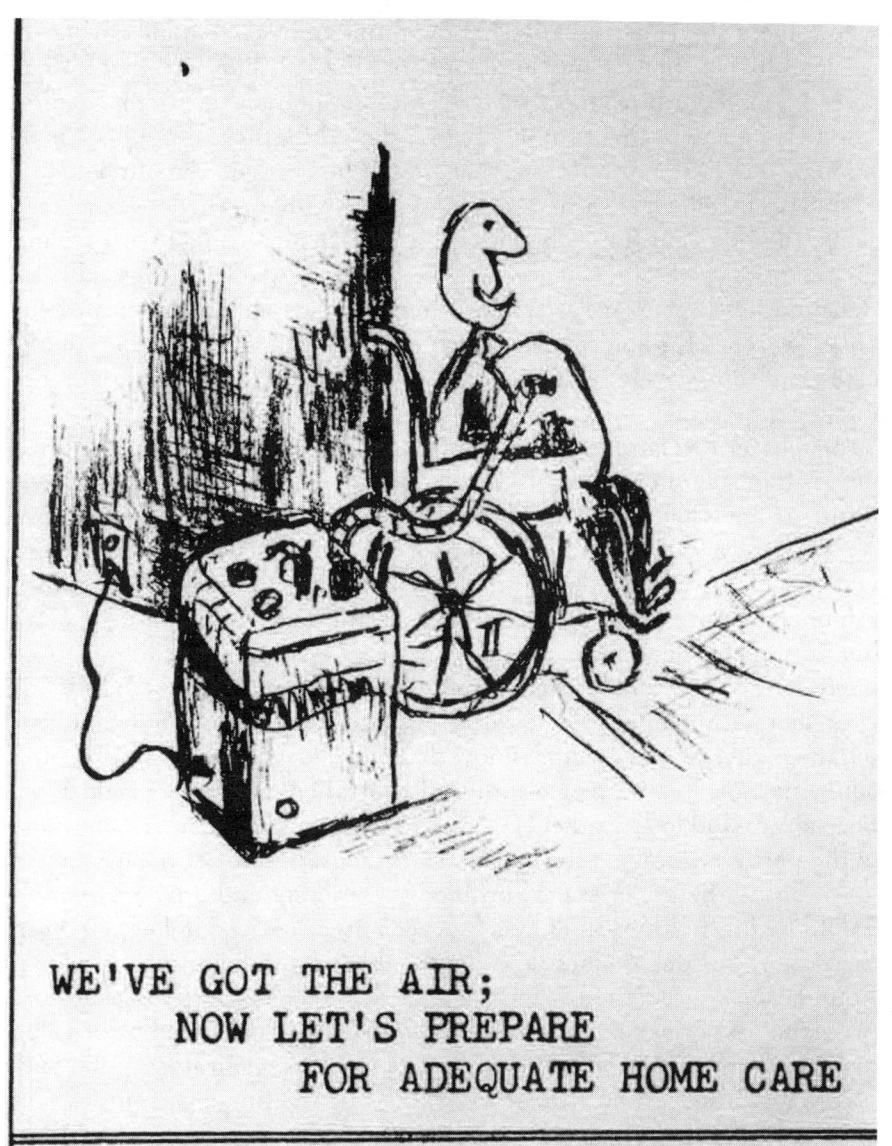

Figure 7. Emmanuel Leplin, artist. Cartoon (rpt. *The Toomey j. Gazette,* Fall-Winter 1959). Courtesy of Rocky Leplin.

who remain single can still live happy, fulfilling lives, that masturbation is a healthy practice for impaired and able-bodied alike, and that for impaired people with partners who wish to maintain a satisfying sex life, "anything goes. In this completely private world, there are no rights or wrongs, there are no traditions that cannot be broken. The ultimate test of success is that an orgasm or sexual climax, with its relief of sexual tensions, should occur for both, with each time an increasing loving feeling for the other."[46] Holbert even speaks approvingly of homosexual relationships (except in cases where same-sex partnering substitutes for failed searches for heterosexual partners), when few mainstream publications of this vintage treated even able-bodied sex in such illuminating, informative terms.

In a letter to a later issue, regular reader-contributor Elbridge Rector details the lack of care he suffers at a public institution. His narrative is bleak—somewhat rambling and purple of prose, but clear enough in describing the abuse he suffered by overworked, uncaring state workers when, evidently, his National Foundation support for private attendance ran out. Rector can barely breathe during the early days at the hospital, due to the absence of the essential rocking bed. He is left alone, unrotated, for hours at a time, then develops a rash when required to lie in his excrement. Shockingly, the letter is followed by an editor's note, informing the audience that Rector is now deceased.[47] Again, such a disturbing confrontation by the tragic indignities of ableist neglect would have been a rare find in any other popular (or even special interest) magazine of the period. Significantly, by the later issues, the *Gazette*'s early motto —"to share the experiences, problems, thoughts and adventures that would be fun to know about each other"—was revised in keeping with these more serious themes, and the trouble portended by the National Foundation's threatened withdrawal of financial support: "to share the problems, experiences, thoughts and adventures that would be of value to know about each other." While the plight of respiratory polio survivors was about to be radically devalued by the financial sources that supported them up this point, this community insisted upon its continuing value and stressed the invaluable connections to be made among each other during this difficult time.

Years of Transformation

In my narrative of the publications issuing from the Warm Springs Foundation, I observed the genre's overgrowth and solidification during the later years of the polio rehab period. We see this phenomenon affecting latter issues of the *Gazette* as well. Though it remained committed, in its instructive content and forthright tone, to total access and equality for the disabled, its very success all but guaranteed a move away from its original grassroots styling—what today we might call a guerilla, underground, or zine format, consciously maintained by alternative publishers. Its articles lengthened, font sizes reduced, pictures crowded in, and pages increased—more than doubling between 1959 (one issue was 39 pages) and 1967 (one issue was 87 pages). One notices similar densification in *Accent on Living*, with increased word and page counts from one issue to the next. Even "Dear Bonnie" fielded more questions and gave longer-winded replies in later columns. Overall, *Accent* had an increasingly legitimized, commercialized feel. The Summer 1970 issue of *Accent* opens with eight pages of advertising; while these continued to feature products designed with the impaired consumer in mind, in many way *Accent on Living* (including its all-purpose title) was less and less distinguishable from any "normal" magazine. Certainly it is the case that for *Gazette* and *Accent* readers more was better in many respects: more information, networking, and humor would always be appreciated; while both publications also eventually gave up their polio-specific identities, new readerships among those spinal cord-injured, generally "handicapped," and otherwise immobilized only increased the size and strength of this interpersonal, cultural, and political coalition. Yet this growth also represents an undeniable loss—of smallness itself, that intimate, direct address that made the earliest issues of these magazines the closest possible textual alternative to a personal friend.

As it transitioned from the 1960s to the 1970s, the *Gazette* maintained an eighty-plus page count but grew in size, from half- to full-sheet and from flat to glossy stock, further legitimizing its presence in the media marketplace, which again had its positive and negative effects. From the early 1970s until 1986, it was an annual publication only, meaning that it no longer played the role of continuous, recurring textual presence within the polio-affected community. Yet despite the large lag between issues, the *Gazette* of the '70s and '80s was a vital source of information, especially, as always, regarding jobs, hobbies, legislation, assistive technologies, and the now bi-annual Post-Polio and Independent Living Conference, held in St. Louis, where the *Gazette* (and editor Gini Laurie) brought the publication from Chagrin Falls in the early 1970s. Most notably, however, the *Gazette* of this era was a vital forum for polio survivors from around the world to share anecdotes and full-length essays—dozens in every issue—related to their health, job, marital, and discrimination experiences. Many of these are accompanied by photos of their authors; other pages feature photo-coverage of *Gazette*-sponsored events, enlivening and personalizing the publication even more; its annual appearance, replete with these many photos, likened the *Gazette* in these decades to an eagerly anticipated college yearbook. In 1986, the *Gazette* became a twice-yearly publication but maintained its large size and reader focus.

Because Laurie had done so much of the editorial work on a volunteer basis, at her passing in 1989, the publication was radically revised. Its new financial needs, as well as its desire to reach its audience more regularly, meant that the *Gazette* of the 1990s and 2000s, renamed *Post-Polio Health*, transformed from an eighty-page, glossy, special interest, reader-oriented semi-annual to a quarterly 6- to 8-page plain-stock newsletter now focused on research on post-polio syndrome.[48] Pitched throughout the mid-1990s toward the "host of doctors, nurses, and physiotherapists who made up a large part" of the earliest *Polio Chronicle*'s circulation, *Post-Polio Health* and its sister publications *Rehabilitation Gazette* (now aimed at a general disability readership) and *Ventilator-Assisted Living* appeared as "industry" newsletters or bulletins—as clinical, professional, and monochromatic as these "house organs" tend to be. One issue of *Post-Polio Health* makes refreshingly casual reference to "Lois in California," who reported finding the Kenny sticks she had been in search of, echoing the chatty, chummy tones of the earliest numbers.[49] Yet overall, the space given to reader news and comment was minimal—sometimes as little as half a column—and one full-length *Post-Polio Health* article devoted to personal narrative was not contributed by a readers but excerpted from Edmund Sass's just-published *Polio's Legacy: An Oral History*.[50] By the late nineties, the focus shifted once more; where almost all of the mid-'90s articles from *Post-Polio Health* and the *Rehabilitation Gazette* were written by MDs, the professionals penning the late-1990s articles carried degrees from the wider spectrum of patient care—for instance MSW (Master's in Social Work) and even CEAP (Certified Employee Assistance Professional). Too, the presence of the lay reader grew once more, both in the number of personal experience essays included and in the focus on cultural themes (e.g., polio fiction, nonfiction, and film reviews) aimed at a mainstream audience. As Joan Headley, the editor who succeeded Laurie, and her staff recognized, however, the internet had effectively taken on the role of regular (even daily or hourly) communication medium for the polio-affected lay community, causing paper versions such as theirs to both downsize and turn their attention elsewhere (personal interview). Yet remarkably, these vibrant early print publications, in their frequent and intensely personal approach to their polio-affected readership, anticipated and effected the connection formation enabled by today's wide spectrum of electronic media.

Conclusion

Indeed, disability media today are more progressive, sophisticated, and numerous than ever; a range of quarterly publications targeting every political and personal demographic has flourished in recent years and expanded (or transformed) into internet formats to reach even wider audiences. *Mainstream Magazine, Mouth—Voice of the Disability Nation*, and especially *Disability Issues* (originally *Together*, founded as a monthly newsletter in 1980) and the pointedly countercultural *Ragged Edge* (originally *Disability Rag*, also begun as a newsletter in 1980) are now well established magazines; newer publications include *New Mobility Magazine* and the web-zine *Disability World*. From Mississippi hails "The Strength Coach," Greg Smith, who hosts a weekly syndicated radio show regarding disability, diversity, and tolerance. On-line discussion groups whose members help each other deal with post-polio syndrome include those featured on *healthboards.com*, *infopolio*, and *P-Life*, among dozens of others. There, information is traded regarding knowledgeable doctors, assistive devices, herbal remedies, and shared symptoms. Frustration and solutions, support and congratulation circulate with each posting. In 2007 All Iowa Reads selected Jeffrey Kluger's *Splendid Solution: Jonas Salk and the Conquest of Polio* (2005) as its communal text and sponsored a website, www.iowapoliostories.org, on which Iowans affected by polio log on and share their recollections. This on-line archive already contains many fascinating accounts, including the tragic story of a young girl whose funeral was held behind a plate glass window, as the family was still in quarantine (Hixon), and a mother's recollection of "sheer terror" in the prevaccine years, when polio "was, of course, on everyone's mind, all the time" (Lieder). Wide-ranging disability blogs include *The Gimp Parade* and *Disability Studies—Temple U*, but the author of a well-regarded children's book, *Small Steps: The Year I Got Polio* (1998), hosts *Peg Kehret's Blog*, which focuses specifically on polio topics.

Certainly, print media continue to serve those who remain outside of internet access, while the web speeds the pace (and thus the significance) of information transmission and personal connection as print forms never can. *SpeciaLiving*, the latest incarnation of *Accent on Living*, is the only surviving publication with specifically polio-related origins, yet I would contend that all of these contemporary serials descend from the polio-specific ur-texts I have considered in this chapter. Topics of concern in contemporary publications—access, equipment, local and world news related to disability issues—reflect those of the *Gazette* and *Accent on Living*; their use of photos, illustrations, and humor increase their appeal and accessibility as did the earliest newsletters from Warm Springs. The interdependence of these publications and disability rights groups with national constituencies (such as the Disability Rights Education and Defense Fund, Justice For All, Not Dead Yet—even Ms. Wheelchair America) is by now complete; it is clear that these publications have been vital to the formation of these groups and that their efforts in turn sustain these texts as ever more vital organs for their respective readerships.

In *Imagined Communities*, Benedict Anderson argues that print culture enabled the concept of nation to replace that of religion not only by explaining and justifying human suffering but by maximizing its market in the shift from Latin to vernacular languages.[51] In this chapter I have examined the vernacular phenomenon of the polio newsletter, which provided those recovering from polio a means by which to recognize themselves when Latinate medical and bureaucratic terminology excluded and alienated them. As polio may be said to have inaugurated the illness pathography genre in nonfiction, so polio happens to have been the first medical issue around which coalesced a genre of serial publication that has nurtured related political movements (disability rights, independent living) of vital historical significance. In tandem with the activism of disabled veterans, who have drawn attention to disability issues since, likely, the American Revolution, and whose media presence (in film, radio, mainstream periodicals, and special-interest magazines) was enormous during this WWII/early postwar period, the editors, reporters, contributors, photographers, artists, and readership for polio newsletters created a mandate and immediately began to fulfill it. In many ways, disability rights serial publication has never departed from the project outlined by Gini Laurie and Sue Williams in their earliest discursive outreachings to their core audience and the able-bodied (and ableist) population beyond: to spread awareness to this wider world that the physically impaired are "young, ambitious, educated . . . energetic and healthy (Yes! Healthy!)" and to build a worldwide network of "valued" persons with impairments through "fun," friendship, information exchange, and united strength.

Conclusion
"The Voice is Still There":
Some Final Notes on Postwar Polio Culture

POSTWAR FILM TREATMENTS OF POLIO ARE AS RARE AND DIVERSE AS literary examples; three that I have encountered share the status of celebrity biography—stories of adults (not children) faced with polio at the thresholds of brilliant careers and caught subsequently between the polio-complicated demands of profession and family. They shed some final light on the questions and themes that have recurred here: the relationship between illness and disability, the gendering of polio and its aftermath, the prevalence of denial and silence in the postwar polio context. In reverse chronological order, Dore Schary's self-adapted stageplay *Sunrise at Campobello* (Vincent J. Donehue, 1960), the film adaptation of opera star Marjorie Lawrence's autobiography, *Interrupted Melody* (Curtis Bernhardt, 1955), and another autobiographical adaptation, *Sister Kenny* (Dudley Nichols, 1946) indicate that the most forthright film treatment of polio is the earliest: in the throes of America's most epidemic years (the immediate postwar period), Hollywood managed to address polio's most frightening, frustrating ramifications in some detail; as it moved further from the crisis (even in 1955, the year the vaccine was proven effective) it tended more and more toward the circumspection that I have identified at many times in this study and that characterized this period as a whole.

The celebrity status of each film's protagonist complicates to some degree the findings of disability film theorists whose observations of nonfamous (or infamous) characters with physical impairments and disfigurations lead these theorists to conclude that such characters are almost always marked as villainous, worthless, pathetic, or, as Martin Norden discerns, "sweet young things whose goodness and innocence are sufficient currency for a one-way ticket out of isolation in the form of a miraculous cure."[1] In the three films considered here, each main character's post-polio status as disabled "spectacle" and as "isolated" in his or her freakish physicality (or even his or her extraordinary ability to compensate) is difficult to separate from what are designated as these public figures' innate talents, courage, and charisma, their personal quests to attain the public stage *before* the onset of polio (or, in the case of Sister Kenny, *because* of polio, as a means to its alleviation). In addition, the historical figure lurking behind each of these biopics calls attention to film's historical tendency to exaggerate, glamorize, or completely misrepresent actual lives; research into FDR and his polio impairment[2] may challenge the authenticity of even well-meaning film treatments such as *Sunrise at Campobello*. Likewise, postwar-era filmgoers, many of whom would have been familiar with the heavy features, white hair, and mannish physique of the real Sister Kenny, would see immediately that little attempt, besides some concession to height and wardrobe, was made by her film biographers to disguise the glamorous Rosalind Russell as any sort of plausible replication of the person she portrayed.

Even one film including a nonfamous, polio-affected "sweet young thing" steps away from the findings of disability theorists in striking ways. In *Leave Her to Heaven* (John M. Stahl, 1946), Gene Tierney (who received an Oscar nomination) plays Ellen, a pathologically possessive young wife who will stop at nothing to have Richard (Cornel Wilde) to herself. This includes sitting by while her future brother-in-law Danny, a teenager with polio-induced paraplegia, loses strength while swimming and drowns in a lake. As we compare the typical formulae by which disabled sympathetic film characters are dispatched (often, as per Norden, through miraculous cure or, as per Longmore, through tragic suicide), this scenario places blame firmly on the beautiful, able-bodied, but evil major character, who pays (with her life) for her crime by the end of the film. Before Danny's demise, Ellen's ableism is plainly on display; she rushes his recovery to crutch-walking so that he can return to boarding school, then frets to the doctors at Warm Springs that "he's a cripple!" when it is determined he would be better off sharing the lakeside home she had plotted to share with Richard alone. Danny's death by drowning indicates perfectly his ball-and-chain status within the film's controlling perspective, again well reflecting typical attitudes toward persons with physical limitations in studio-era Hollywood and to a large extent today, which few films of either period have had the courage to admit.

Meanwhile, most valuable is Norden's comment that (even when considering film treatments of polio-affected international celebrities) mainstream Hollywood films use lighting, set design, editing, and of course the scripts themselves "to suggest a physical or symbolic separation of disabled characters from the rest of society."[3] Because one example considered here (FDR) belongs to American aristocracy, I am inspired by Norden's argument to nuance the concept of "society" to refer to not only people in general (the masses, if you will) but society as social class, to consider briefly the way in which each character indeed falls from society, the class-peers with whom s/he associated early in the film, once polio strikes. For Marjorie Lawrence, the onset of polio signals her self-imposed exile from professional engagement and the glamour of New York, just as Norden has indicated. For both the blue-blooded Roosevelt and the middle-class Elizabeth Kenny, their respective societal dictates emphasized privacy and circumspection—reserve and gentility for Roosevelt, dutiful hospital servitude then respectable marriage for Nurse Kenny. Their encounters with polio cause both to violate these dictates, enmesh themselves with great numbers of the lower orders (i.e., a very different kind of society), to the horror of their class-conscious home circles. While polio eventually enables both FDR and Sister Kenny toward maximum societal integration (for FDR, this is with both his cohort at Warm Springs and the voters of America; for Sister Kenny, this is with the polio-affected of the world), both turn against (and are in part turned against by) their original social environments and all three polio protagonists tumble (either temporarily or permanently) from their elevated social ranks, just as polio causes the affected characters in each film to stumble and fall. As is the case with many of the polio texts analyzed throughout this study, here each film metaphorizes polio-related disability in ways that both contain and enlarge its significance: FDR and Marjorie Lawrence reinhabit their respective social contexts with polio-related impairment in tow; Sister Kenny remains resolutely outside a society depicted ultimately as snobbish, narrow-minded, and hypocritical anyway.

Sister Kenny's black and white photography complements the grimness of its heroine's often losing battle with polio; the color-drunk renditions of Marjorie Lawrence's story (filmed in glorious CinemaScope) and FDR's earliest years with polio (in equally impressive Technicolor) are operatic, melodramatic, and triumphant. The clear-cut victories concluding these latter two films—both end, nearly identically with the hero/ine rising from a chair and walking unassisted at a moment of triumphant return to the public stage — contrast with the somewhat hollow victory of Sister Kenny, who receives the acclaim of the children and families helped by her therapeutic methods but remains a figure on the margin of the medical profession. While career threatens the bonds both between FDR (played by Ralph Bellamy) and his wife and mother and between Lawrence (brought haughtily to life by Eleanor Parker) and her adoring fiancé, in fact polio brings together family members in both cases, who reject the prospect of success for the hero/ine before illness, then see a successfully resumed career as a well-deserved reward following the rehabilitation phase. Perhaps much truer to life, especially for many polio-affected women, Nurse Kenny loses her romantic prospects to polio, when her devotion to helping sick children causes her fiancé to walk out of her life. She ends the film alone, despite being surrounded by the adulating "people." Of the three, Sister Kenny is the film character uninfected with polio herself, yet whose story is in many ways most tragic.

Before polio strikes each narrative (in Lawrence's, this is well past the halfway point) its lead character struggles with the same dilemma: whether to pursue a career (in politics, opera, or nursing) or succumb to the influences of spouse and family. One would think this a nonexistent problem for Roosevelt (or any man in this period), who would have been encouraged to marry, father children, and succeed in business without conflict of interest. But in fact Roosevelt's high standing and tremendous wealth ill-suit him (at least according to his aristocratic mother) to business doings of any kind, much less to a tawdry role in national politics. Eleanor (Greer Garson, who got an Oscar nomination for the role) is more supportive of Franklin's pre-polio immersion in public service but fears the larger role she herself might have to play, as well as the prospect of having to share him with a large, anonymous constituency. Much less surprising is the fork-in-the-road met by the female leads. Both rising star Marjorie Lawrence and talented Nurse Kenny are delivered an ultimatum by their loving fiancés: marriage and motherhood with themselves *or* professional success — never both.[4] While Sister Kenny toys with the idea of permanent professional sidelining, successive polio outbreaks summon and resummon her, until her romantic relationship dissolves. Meanwhile Marjorie gives up a South American tour and a debut at Covent Garden when her beloved Dr. Walker (Glenn Ford) tires of waiting.

Significantly, Marjorie's failure to keep this wedding vow leads immediately to her (literal) downfall; during rehearsals in South America she collapses from polio, at which point it is her new husband's turn to give up his career to nurse her back to health. Her proud manner as a successful performer is a debilitating—and fascinating—character flaw as she faces the prospect of rehabilitation. At first she is cowardly and vain about "crawling" in public; even after moving from bed to wheelchair to piano bench—where she learns elatedly that "the voice is still there"—she is an emotional invalid terrified to sing in public, threatening her family's finances and her husband's ability to resume his obstetrical career. While her biography provides a different timeline, the film returns Marjorie to the operatic stage after she is inspired to sing to a ward full of recovering GIs, many of them wheelchair-using like herself, and taken on a performance tour for soldiers in every far-flung outpost.[5] As Martin Norden has observed, films about wounded soldiers and disabled veterans were ubiquitous in this period, keeping the issue of disability in the cultural forefront. Polio borrowed into and reinforced that public presence on multiple other occasions and does so once again in this film. Norden also describes films' tendency to "isolate disabled characters from . . . each other," to "divide-and-quarantine" their disabled minority figures,[6] and the exceptional nature of this moment tends to prove his rule: Marjorie's interaction with veteran wheelchair-users is the film's turning point; their convocation in the hospital setting is a pivotal and powerful visual image. While once Marjorie's husband fought her professional success, her triumphant return to opera is a victory for him as well as her—just as FDR's taking the podium to nominate Al Smith in the 1924 democratic convention is witnessed with glowing pride by both Eleanor and his overbearing mother. Roosevelt in this film observes about himself (as have many biographers since) that he (like Marjorie Lawrence) was too proud and too frivolous to be worthy of history-making in his youthful, pre-polio days. For both Lawrence and Roosevelt, polio is correctively character-building even as it hobbles both physically for life.

Sunrise at Campobello comments poignantly on the frustrations and fatigue induced by Roosevelt's abelist environment. Still adjusting to his constant chair occupation, Roosevelt is exasperated by visitors from the worlds of business and politics, who insensitively pace around the room instead of sitting quietly as he must; in a bit of tragicomedy, a group of his (literal) supporters rush him on a stretcher to a train, just as a panting press corps arrives on the scene. Having whisked his disability from the public eye with a mere whisker of time to spare, Franklin greets the reporters merrily, seated of course, from a window in the train, then falls asleep in exhaustion as soon as the train leaves the station. For me, the film's most effective scene involves the sort of "crawling" that Marjorie Lawrence refuses to attempt in her own story: in his early convalescent stage, Roosevelt flings himself cheerfully from his chair and inches his way up a long staircase, treating his wife and business manager, Louis Howe, to his trademark wave and smile as he disappears at the top. In response, Eleanor and Louis betray the ableist gaze of horror. For them, this is no moment of triumph but a humiliating apprehension of the depths to which this great man has sunk. They are hurt and embarrassed on his behalf; the film is halfhearted in condemning this waste of unsolicited emotional energy, feeling Eleanor's "pain" too much, yet modern viewers may observe and learn from the sharp contrast between Roosevelt's mobilizing aplomb and his loved ones' pointlessly tragic reaction.

In *Interrupted Melody* Marjorie is prettily arranged on a Florida beach when she attracts the attention of two wolfish morning joggers, who attempt to pick her up, then dash off when they spy her wheelchair. Later, she panics and retreats from a concert performance with the Florida Philharmonic when she learns that the audience has come not to "hear" her but to "see" her (i.e., gaze at her freakish physical situation). Her triumphant first steps at film's end are artfully choreographed and supported by the gorgeous atmospherics of Wagner's *Tristan und Isolde*, staged entirely around Marjorie's need to remain seated. As she rises painfully and drapes herself grievously over Tristan's corpse during the stirring finale, it is clear that this blocking was her own willful idea, as husband, director, and cast members look on from the wings with a mixture of shock, concern, anger, adulation, and love. Despite what may be perceived as a hammy performance and cheesy theatrics by modern viewers, it is a moving conclusion whose implied thesis is that Marjorie's impairment has given this classic love story power and significance it never had. Not surprisingly, *Interrupted Melody* received the most Oscar nominations of the three considered here.[7]

Despite the gains sought after in both films, both make their concessions to the cultural mandate of silencing polio discourse—literally by refraining from using the term or showing in any detail the disease's damaging effects. In each film, a single reference to the main character's diagnosis seems sufficient: In consultation with the doctor, Eleanor exclaims over "Infantile!" in horrified disbelief and never mentions it again. She employs the 1920s-era term for polio (i.e., infantile paralysis) that ensures the film's historical accuracy while sparing mid-century audiences from the more familiar yet still unnerving term polio. FDR himself never hears the diagnosis or uses the word. Similarly, in her post-acute stage, Marjorie awakes beautifully, as from a long nap—often one is in too much pain to sleep during polio's earliest phases—and is told by her husband only that she is "pretty sick." Again, it is he and the doctor who speak in frank terms, while Marjorie is spared having to confront her situation at the level of language. Not surprisingly, *Interrupted Melody*'s promotional material shares the linguistic diffidence: "Crippling paralysis" is the term of choice for the liner notes to the Turner/MGM laserdisc and video, while the original trailer barely indicates a medical problem.

In sharp contrast, *Sister Kenny* calls constant attention to the name of polio and its specific clinical manifestations. In an early scene, bush nurse Sister Kenny visits the home of a young girl whose painful cries have her parents in a panic. When the blanket is pulled back, she sees the arched back and bent knees of early polio contracture and talks at length—and with moving interest—about the pulling and pushing muscles causing this deformity. Though she must telegraph medical authorities in the city to learn that these symptoms mean polio, she knows instinctively that moist heat will provide the necessary relief and wraps the child in boiled, wrung-out strips of wool. At last the girl is eased by this treatment and falls asleep, with parents and audiences relieved by the silence that follows the persistent, heartbreaking whining of the last several scenes. Hopes are again dashed when the child looks well but still cannot move, and while full recovery comes too easily—with a few moments of pushing, stroking, and pep-talking, the child is kicking again—this victory withers on the vine of medical orthodoxy when Sister Kenny's near-perfect record of treatment in the back country is dismissed by city physicians.

Though finally given "hopeless" cases to straighten and mobilize as best she can, Sister Kenny longs to apply her hot packs to acute cases; her repeated requests are denied with the vehemence leveled against child-abusers. Much of the film dwells on humiliating accusations of quackery that, while roundly denounced by the film's perspective, stop the heroine in her tracks. Repeated frustration takes its physical toll, as Russell grays her hair and changes out of the fetching dresses of early scenes into the baggy, unflattering suits famously worn by the real Sister Kenny. Ironically, her increasingly "professionalized" appearance is a reaction to, and a useless antidote against, the exclusion from the profession she has faced since the beginning. At last receiving a modicum of support in the United States, she is invited to Minnesota where a hospital's medical staff (entirely male) finally acknowledges her remarkable success.

In contrast to the final scenes of the other two films, however, Sister Kenny's triumphant taking of the stage—a seminar she conducts for a large audience of receptive physicians—is deeply marred. Instead of a spouse standing supportively by to witness her moment in the sun, she learns moments earlier that a beloved mentor has passed away. Emotionally devastated, she commences her presentation anyway, when a voice over the loudspeaker announces yet again that in the latest medical studies Sister Kenny's methods are deemed unscientific and therefore unsupportable. She is immediately turned upon by the more skeptical in her audience; although she retains the support of others, this is hardly a moment of universal acclaim. As the camera pulls back and the credits roll, Sister Kenny moves from the hospital to the streets, returning to the role of beloved, "backward" bush nurse that she once zealously chose for herself but that has defeated her during all later stages of her career. Receiving bouquets from a sea of grateful children, they join a rising chorus of "Happy Birthday"; of all things, she turns another unwed year older on this same day.

How do these three remarkable films complete our understanding of "the voice" (and of course, for film, "the look") of polio in postwar America? From the first chapter, the ringing silences surrounding polio have been as instructive as have those voices that did speak out. I have defined this silent cultural response in various ways: as a literal absence or infrequency of word or image in popular textual genres at key moments in the postwar polio timeline; as an anxious or diffident circling-around that fails to resolve in head-on, therapeutic confrontation; as elaborate gestures of denial (understatement) *or* melodramatization (overstatement) that are as effusive and noisy as a March of Dimes parade but that profit the cause much less. Yet as the "perfect" textual response to polio is rare (or nonexistent), so the great majority of written replies that miss the mark are less productively read as failures than as naturally occurring, richly loaded indicators of the shape polio anxieties and sorrows took in the cultural imagination at this time. Likewise the films considered here include elements of silence and speech, and in the visual register elision and representation, suggesting the mix of confrontation and denial that characterized many polio memoirs of that same era and may have proved most therapeutic to postwar, anxiety-ridden audiences.

As visual narratives, these films involve a relationship between image and language that recalls the remarkable look of two very different kinds of polio texts: the postwar women's magazines whose lush illustrations and cheery domestic photography often jarred against the grim, vague, or contradictory language contained in the article proper; and the polio rehabilitation center newsletter, whose combination of words and pictures sent specific messages to its audience with respect to a grassroots versus commercial ethos, assimilation versus advocacy, and the elite spa versus the college campus versus the virtual community center. Above, I contrasted *Sister Kenny*'s black-and-white tones to the vibrant color displays of the other two films; the contrast between realistic (both "black and white," *and* "grey area") treatments of polio and their more escapist counterparts has been a structuring opposition throughout my inquiry. In the magazines, creative, colorful, romanticized layout enabled editors to frame, marginalize, or minimize polio's most disturbing details; at the rehab centers, each newsletter's pictorial style and all-around visual presentation—elegant, slapdash, free-form, densely shaded—almost always coincided with its verbal content and disability perspective. While the newsletters relied almost entirely upon black and white photography and cheaply reproduced line drawing, yet they provided a total spectrum of mood, aesthetic, and cultural and political conservatism and progressivism in their remarkable array of visual styles and deployments.

As discussed above, these films draw upon the historical proportions of their famous subjects to lend significance to the films themselves and to historicize the meaning of polio in the postwar era. Thus the films help us to think about the interimplicated meanings of history that have circulated throughout this study: the historic as the past, the historic as the actual (as opposed to the mythic or fictional), and the historic as the temporal (as opposed to the static or timeless). These midcentury films lack the long perspective of contemporary polio novels, which place the polio experience firmly and often instructively within the confines of the American past; yet the protagonist of each struggles, and in-part succeeds, with putting polio into his or her personal past while at the same time relying upon polio's hard reality to substantiate and dimensionalize an ambivalent career and superfluous character pre-polio, to enlarge upon the very historical significance each continues to be credited with: without polio, would Sister Kenny have ever left the Australian back country? Would Roosevelt have been the president he was? Would Marjorie Lawrence's career have had the same memorable poignancy, supported to some extent by the Hollywood treatment it received, which is ordinarily accorded only to those opera luminaries (e.g., Enrico Caruso) facing early death or severe physical crisis? As with many of the polio memoirists considered throughout this study, polio is read as an ultimately constructive "reality check" that literally and metaphorically transforms the protagonist into a much more thoughtful, centered, and down-to-earth individual. Finally, while each polio-affected film protagonist is on his or her feet in the final scene, not one "walks away from polio," as did the protagonists of some of the more fortunate writers of polio memoirs and novels. The literal stance taken by these lead characters (and hence by the films themselves) suggests the sort of "triumph" over polio the Hollywood filmgoer was assumed to require in this era, yet stands against notions of easy victory by indicating simultaneously the pain, sacrifice, and politics involved in each of these ultimately false steps.

None of the film protagonists is portrayed as requiring respirator assistance at any point post-polio, so the radical reconfigurations of gender and sexuality roles on display in various of the iron-lung memoirs and novels discussed in this study are not on view in these films. Yet these films—especially the two featuring female subjects—reflect instructively upon the issues of sex, gender, and sexuality that have preoccupied this study and those of feminist disability scholars whose ideas have been influential here. Polio threatened the careers of Franklin Roosevelt and Marjorie Lawrence and enabled the career of Elizabeth Kenny; the polio memoirs (and a few of the novels) combine these plotlines, since a striking majority of their authors were writers before polio and/or pursued writing (or academic) careers, whose minimal physical requirements suited them well, following polio. Of course the correlation between "polio" and "professor" or "professional writer" is much lower than that between "polio text" and the writerly inclination that affected various polio survivors even before or aside from their being presented with this remarkable subject to write about. Yet the coincidence between authorial intent and the realization of the finished written work, as this is enabled by the onset of polio, accounts for many of the more upbeat subplots and happy endings of polio narratives considered here. Certainly, less affected polio narrators (and novel characters) resume other kinds of work; especially the male ones are allowed to do so, while the female memoirists and fictional figures face the financial and emotional crisis of "livelihood"—who will care for them and their children once the fiancé or husband disappears and state-sponsored support ebbs away?

Interestingly, none of the memoirists considered in this study indicates that s/he writes to survive; always the polio memoir comes from fortunate-enough circumstances of familial or institutional financial support, allowing the writer the leisure to tell his or her story on his or her own terms and achieve more a sense of professional accomplishment than vital remuneration from the completed task. As a 2:1 majority of polio memoirists considered in chapter 2 (and as it turns out another 2:1 majority of the polio novelists considered in chapter 3) are men, the indication once more is that many polio-affected women lack the necessary financial and personal security to turn to writing as a creative and compensatory option. Not surprisingly, the three polio biopics analyzed in this conclusion are about exceptional people, stars in their respective fields portrayed by Hollywood stars; these exceptions to the rule, however, require us to consider the rule itself, the ordinary polio-affected man or woman in midcentury America whose personal, professional, and marital situations were often much more gravely threatened by the difficulties caused by polio. Also, true to what some of the memoirs and much of the feminist disability scholarship indicates, the marital outcomes of these polio-affected film protagonists are typical: the male character never faces for a moment the prospect of losing his family or financial standing, the female character who is able to "walk away from polio" saves her marriage thereby, and the female character who refuses to do so is left alone at film's end.

If these films, as Hollywood productions, represent the most popular, influential, and thus also ideologically enmeshed of all the polio genres considered in this study, they yet share a place in my conceptual chronology with the least "popular" (i.e., most unprofessionalized) genre in this study—the polio newsletter or magazine. For like these in-house, in-group serial publications, the films considered here situate their famous protagonists (and admiring audiences) before the onset of polio, then present both with the experience of permanent association with it, even as each film itself draws to a close: fifteen years after his death, for instance, Roosevelt "lives on" for filmgoers of 1960 whose viewing of this film might have reinforced (or introduced for the first time) the understanding that as a beloved and immortal historical figure, Roosevelt and his physical impairment will always be with us, just as the impairment itself accompanied Roosevelt to his last day. Such representations, which enable both the physically impaired and the able-bodied mainstream to contemplate the reality and the significance of the ongoingness of impaired living, are those I have described throughout this study as unflinching, historically accurate, and therapeutic. While all of the polio textual genres considered here offer something of this experience to their readerships, it is the genre of the rehab newsletter that stands for me as most exemplary. For their respective enclaves of circulation, the arrival of each new issue was as eagerly anticipated as next Friday night's film; as seemingly trivial and escapist as the splashiest Technicolor musical or melodrama, polio rehab newsletters performed the serious work of recovery (of body and identity) *through* their focus on the "frivolous" and "meaningless"—redefining and revaluing what the able-bodied mainstream had written off as insignificant, as the disability rights movement has continued to do since the polio era. Amidst the wealth of fascinating silences constituting the cultural response to polio from the postwar period to the present day, this remarkable voice, among others, "is still there," and this study has sought to distinguish these, and forge connections among them as they constitute polio's American textual legacy.

Notes

INTRODUCTION

1. Robert F. Hall, *Through the Storm: A Polio Story* (St. Cloud, MN: North Start Press of St. Cloud, 1990), 4.

2. Ibid., 20.

3. See Hugh Gregory Gallagher, *FDR's Splendid Deception* (Arlington, VA: Vandamere Press, 1994); Tony Gould, *A Summer Plague: Polio and Its Survivors* (New Haven: Yale University Press, 1995); Jeffrey Kluger, *Splendid Solution: Jonas Salk and the Conquest of Polio* (New York: G.P. Putnam's Sons, 2005); David M. Oshinsky, *Polio: An American Story* (New York, Oxford University Press, 2005); Naomi Rogers, *Dirt and Disease: Polio Before FDR* (Rutgers: Rutgers University Press, 1992); Marc Shell, *Polio and its Aftermath: The Paralysis of Culture* (Cambridge, MA: Harvard University Press, 2005); Jane S. Smith, *Patenting the Sun: Polio and the Salk Vaccine* (New York: Anchor/Doubleday, 1990); and Daniel J. Wilson, *Living with Polio: The Epidemic and Its Survivors* (Chicago: University of Chicago Press, 2005). Shell and Wilson both interpret texts, as I do in this work, Wilson from a specifically historical perspective. Shell is a literary critic, not a historian like Wilson, although his work is itself partly a memoir of his own polio experience, and his text selection differs in large part from mine.

4. Smith, *Patenting the Sun*, 42.

5. I appreciate Lorenzo Wilson Milam's formulation of polio's terrifying randomness: "a captious disease: like a tornado, dipping down to lay waste to some parts of the land of the body; then skipping over other parts completely." Milam, *The Cripple Liberation Front Marching Band Blues* (San Diego: Mho & Mho Works, 1984), 44.

6. Oshinsky, *American Story*, 9.

7. Smith, *Patenting the Sun*, 42.

8. G. Thomas Couser, *Recovering Bodies: Illness, Disability, and Life Writing*. Introduction Nancy Mairs (Madison: University of Wisconsin Press, 1997), 5.

9. Arthur W. Frank *The Wounded Storyteller: Body, Illness, and Ethics* (Chicago: University of Chicago Press, 1995), 75–96.

10. Smith, *Patenting the Sun*, 39. See also Rogers, *Dirt and Disease*.

11. While medical historians continue to ponder whether Roosevelt's paralysis was in fact due to Guillaume-Barré syndrome and not polio, due among other reasons to the extreme rarity of adult infections in the 1920s, his role as a "polio survivor" is key to the story of polio in America. I read FDR's "polio" as a medical and lay perception with vital historical significance, if nothing else.

12. Oshinsky, *American Story*, 51.

13. Ibid., 5.

14. Rosemarie Garland Thomson, *Extraordinary Bodies: Figuring Physical Disability in American Culture and Literature* (New York: Columbia University Press, 1997), 10–11.

15. I refer here to Helen Hayes, who introduced a polio memoir by Eleanor Chappell, *On the Shoulders of Giants: The Bea Wright Story* (discussed in chapter 2). Eleanor Roosevelt wrote the foreword to Turnley Walker's *Roosevelt and the Warm Springs Story* and was a noted advice columnist of women's magazines of the period.

1. "A Battle of Silence"

1. André Fontaine, "The Town that Fought For Its Kids," *Redbook* (July 1950), 46.

2. Ibid., 77.

3. An index search indicates that from 1948 to 1955 *Life* magazine ran 32 articles related to polio, *Time* 72, and *Newsweek* 78; by contrast *Ladies Home Journal* published only seven pieces during that same period with *Better Homes and Gardens*, *Good Housekeeping*, and *McCall's* each presenting four. *Redbook*, aimed at a more mixed audience, departed from this trend with exposés on "quack" doctors, tainted produce, the Kinsey report, and corrupt politicians; the notorious anti-momist ideologue Philip Wylie was a regular contributor who kept world issues like communism and the atom bomb before his audience, when traditional women's magazines dealt only fitfully with the issue of communism and carried on as if the bomb had never been invented. The tradition of overlooking polio continues today in, of all places, scholarly treatments of this period: neither Elaine Tyler May nor Steven Mintz and Susan Kellogg make more than passing reference to the issue in their analysis of women's postwar culture. Kathryn Black points out that David Halberstam's massive, supposedly definitive chronicle, *The Fifties*, is utterly silent. May, *Homeward Bound: American Families in the Cold War Era* (New York: Basic Books, 1988); Mintz and Kellogg, *Domestic Revolutions: A Social History of American Family Life* (New York: Free Press, 1988); Black, *In the Shadow of Polio: A Personal and Social History* (Reading, MA: Addison-Wesley, 1996), 262. See also Shell, Marc. *Polio and its Aftermath: The Paralysis of Culture*, Cambridge, MA: Haarvaard University Press, 2005.

4. Nancy A. Walker, *Shaping Our Mothers' World: American Women's Magazines* (Jackson: University of Mississippi Press, 2000), 49.

5. Ibid., 151.

6. One editor's column for *Good Housekeeping* praises its secretarial staff yet undermines the gesture with its patronizing opinions about the secretaries' "pothooks in the notebooks" (whatever this means), "silly hats," and the sight of "a covey of them hashing over a weekend." "The Girls in the Front Office," *Good Housekeeping* (July 1952), 14. My argument in this chapter counters the perspective voiced by David Reed, who posits that the women's magazine readership itself "was not interested in mental health or other tendentious topics. It just wanted more of what they had always enjoyed in the past and wanted it cheaply." Reed, *The Popular Magazine in Britain and the United States, 1880–1960* (London: British Library, 1997), 204.

7. Despite the phobia regarding polio and other controversial subjects, there is evidence elsewhere of successful interference by the magazines' directors in market and government affairs. See Walker, *Shaping*, 61, 64. On the women's health advocacy accomplished by *Journal* editors Bruce and Beatrice Gould, see Kathleen L. Endres and Therese L. Lueck, eds., *Women's Periodicals in the United States: Consumer Magazines* (Westport, CT: Greenwood Press, 1995). On the career of pure food crusader Harvey W.

Wiley, chief chemist at the USDA and later bureau director at *Good Housekeeping*, see Frank Luther Mott, *A History of American Magazines*, 5 vols (Cambridge, MA: Harvard University Press, 1938–68) and "Harvey W. Wiley: Pioneer Consumer Activist," *Good Housekeeping* (February 1990): 146. *Good Housekeeping* also banned cigarette advertising in 1952, a dozen years before the first surgeon general warnings, while Susanne Williams, director of Consumer and Reader Services for the magazine, notes that today lucrative ads for dietary supplements are frequently turned down. Williams, personal interview, January 21, 2004.

8. Jane S. Smith notes that among the groups receiving separate appeals from the National Foundation were the National Council of Catholic Women, the National Council of Negro Women, and the National Federation of Women's Clubs (Smith 85). An especially telling quote regarding "the high level of parental support" comes from the Foundation director of the Women's Division: "They thought it was their vaccine! They had done so much volunteer work, each of them felt she was a majority stockholder!" (Smith 87). See also Margaret Hickey, ed., "Have We Won the Fight Against Polio?" (December 1954): 25ff.

9. See David M. Oshinsky, *Polio: An American Story* (New York: Oxford University Press, 2005), 30–33.

10. May, *Homeward Bound*; Mintz and Kellogg, *Domestic Revolutions*.

11. Lionel White, "The Girl Who Never Gave Up," *Redbook* (June 1952): 46ff.

12. Margaret Clark, "Polio is Being Defeated," *McCall's* (January 1953), 48ff.

13. See Hickey. Yet indirect references continue in the post-vaccine period; an item entitled "Conquering a New Disease" describes a form of blindness affecting premature babies that has likely been a problem for decades, if not centuries but has been newly entered into the queue to be "conquered," now that the "old" menace (polio, of course) has been put to rest. (Peter Briggs, "Conquering a New Disease" [May 1955], 133).

14. Clark, "Polio is Being Defeated," 107. Finally, in the March 1954 issue of *McCall's*, the optimistic tone of Hart Van Riper, M.D., medical director of the National Foundation, is warranted. His brief but detailed feature, "What You Should Know about Polio Prevention" regards nothing about avoiding swimming pools or staying rested, but the exciting vaccine trials then under way. (Hart Van Riper, M.D., "What You Should Know about Polio Prevention," *McCall's* [March 1954]: 136–37.)

15. William F. McDermott, "The House that Kindness Built," *McCall's* (August 1953): 36ff.

16. Ibid., 124.

17. Richard Frey, "Your Child's Camp and POLIO," *Good Housekeeping* (May 1950): 54.

18. Ibid.

19. Ibid.

20. Ibid., 55.

21. Maxine Davis, "First Complete Handbook on Infantile Paralysis," *Good Housekeeping* (August 1950): 56.

22. Ibid., 200.

23. Ibid., 201.

24. Ibid.

25. Ibid., 202.

26. John Berger, *Ways of Seeing* (London: British Broadcasting Corporation and Penguin Books, [1972] 1977), 151–52.

27. "Polio Pledge," *Redbook* (September 1952): 86.
28. "If Polio Strikes My Home," *Ladies Home Journal* (June 1952): 86.
29. Fontaine, "Town," 76.
30. Ibid., 77.
31. Kay McNeill, as told to Isabella Taves, "10 Million Women are in Love with my Husband," *McCall's* (July 1951): 32ff.
32. Helen Hayes, "I Learned to Live Through Heartbreak," *McCall's* (July 1952): 34ff.
33. "Mother, Beware," *McCall's* (October 1952): 22.
34. Sylvia F. Porter, "What to do in a PANIC," *Good Housekeeping* (June 1950): 54ff+.
35. Felix Charles, M.D., "I'm Proud of My Lies," *McCall's* (January 1952): 89.
36. Kate Holliday, "The Disease that Imitates POLIO," *McCall's* (August 1952): 42ff.
37. Arthur Gordon, "The Doctor Speaks Out," *McCall's* (February 1953): 17ff.
38. Leo Smollar, M.D., "It Won't Kill You!," *Redbook* (May 1952): 21ff. In a turn that surprises not at all, Smollar's "mildly neurotic" patients turn out to be primarily women, and the positioning of the (hysterical) female patient in these sensational accounts that end up being about "nothing" is a nearly universal occurrence. Certainly, the Q&A format of many of these magazines' medical columns assumes a female interlocutor whose half-dozen or more urgent fears of essentially minor illnesses are simultaneously alleviated and invalidated by the answering authority's brief, blithe remarks. On the other end of this catch-22, women with truly serious conditions were often "shielded" from the truth, so that even grave situations were made into "nothing" by the collusion of doctor and husband.
39. Isabella Taves, "Jane Froman: Courage Unlimited," *McCall's* (May 1952): 30ff.
40. In a striking departure from this trend, Herman N. Bundesen addresses "Polio" in his monthly column for *Ladies Home Journal*, "Protecting Your Child from . . ." In this straightforward, well-rounded comment, Dr. Bundesen touches on all of the issues of concern at that time—crowded theaters and swimming areas, hygiene, tonsillectomy, warning signs, and so on. He concurs with others that movies and swimming *are* okay, if there are no polio outbreaks in the area, reassuring advice that yet might have confused parents who wished to play it absolutely safe. In addition, the singularity of this example raises several questions: once Dr. Bundesen had made these pronouncements for the *Journal* back in 1950, was the issue not to be revisited in any of the doctors' columns in these several publications in the many subsequent months until the polio vaccine? Was polio simply a victim of an editorial "once is enough" policy to keep readers from becoming bored or, conversely, hysterical with fear? (Norman H. Bundesen, M.D., "Protecting Your Child From Polio," *Ladies Home Journal* [July 1950]: 133–34.)
41. Irma Simonton Black's monthly column for *Redbook* provides an example of the hortatory tone one discerns in such writings. Her exclamatory titles—"Don't Fence Me In!" (about "playpen overuse") and "Let the Kids Cook!"—and texts that insist much more than suggest presume an audience of inept and negligent mothers. (Irma Simonton Black, "Don't Fence Me In!" *Redbook* [November 1952], 73; Irma Simonton Black, "Let The Kids Cook!" *Redbook* [October 1952], 93). As Walker has noted, the editorial tone of mid-century women's magazines "made [it] clear that women were particularly in need of expert advice." (Walker 152) Meanwhile, Marjorie Ferguson attributes the very existence of women's magazines to "an implicit assumption shared between editors and publishers that a female sex that is at best unconfident and at worst incompetent, 'needs' or 'wants' to be instructed, rehearsed, or brought up to date." (Marjorie Fergu-

son, *Forever Feminine: Women's Magazines and the Cult of Femininity* [London: Heinemann, 1983]: 2.)

42. Marie Killilea, "She Lived a Miracle," *Ladies Home Journal* (August 1952): 36ff.
43. Floyd Miller, "Camp is *Good* For 'Em!," *Redbook* (May 1952): 52ff.
44. "A Boy's Summer," *McCall's* (July 1954): 26–29.
45. Dr. John Fitch Landon, "The Questions You Ask the Doctor about Summer Problems," *McCall's* (July 1953): 95.
46. If the *Journal* cover from July 1951 is more moving yet, it is because an unadorned photograph with a similar theme replaces the sentimentalized illustrations of the other examples. In the photo, a girl of about three poses with her back to the camera at the water's edge. She looks off to her left, as if in search of something, and her simple stance conveys a quiet seriousness, not silliness or joy. A wide angle has been employed, so that the expanse of crashing sea is all around her, and so that "Mom," represented by the camera's perspective, seems too far away to protectively reach her daughter in time. Despite the attempt to capture an image serene or inviting, this child seems to have been abandoned at the shore, and abandoned to the dangers that might lurk just beyond.
47. While the guilty parents and brave children I envision here would primarily constitute a family dealing with a polio-stricken child, even two true-life stories of adult polio survivors play out this dynamic of reversed generational roles. In "Year of Conquest over Polio" emphasis is laid on the upheaval caused by Olga's long polio-induced absence from her family. After months of "sitting down on the job" of motherhood, she is distressed when her children run to a nanny for comfort and advice, and worries over what the months of separation into the homes of different family friends will mean later for her four young children. (Neal G. Stuart, "Year of Conquest over Polio," *Ladies Home Journal* [October 1956]: 187ff.) In "I Can Do Anything But Walk," Grace Grissom's eldest daughter (9 or 10 at most) takes on a supportive role during her mother's bout with polio, doing the legwork necessary to nurse her father through a feverish illness, helping the other kids to mind, and anticipating her mother's needs; a touching detail informs us that "Sylvia has been giving herself a nightly bath since she was five. When she was younger she used to sing all the while she was in the water so that I would know she was all right." (Grace Grissom, as told to Jhan and June Robbins, "I Can Do Anything but Walk," *Redbook* [October 1955], 100).
48. Joe McCarthy, "Frothingham," *Good Housekeeping* (July 1950), 60.
49. Ibid., 222.
50. Maggie Miller,"The Fair-Weather Kind," *McCall's* (February 1952), 102.
51. Vera Henry, "Free as a Gull," *Redbook* (April 1952), 86.
52. Miller, "The Fair-Weather Kind," 102.
53. Henry, "Free as a Gull," 86.
54. Laura Owen Miller, "Dangerous Summer," *McCall's* (May 1952): 39.
55. Ibid., 80.
56. Ibid.
57. Ibid., 74.
58. Ibid.
59. Ibid., 78.
60. Ibid., 82.
61. Ibid.
62. Ibid., 86.

63. Ibid.
64. Ibid., 88.
65. Ibid., 82.
66. Ibid., 80.
67. See also Shell, 175.
68. Suzanne Kaufman, "Summer Bachelor," *McCall's* (September 1950), 28.
69. Ibid.
70. Ibid., 90.
71. Ibid.
72. Ibid.
73. Ibid.
74. See Bundesen.
75. Laura Owen Miller, "Dangerous Summer," 90.
76. Ibid., 98.
77. Ibid.
78. Ibid., 101.
79. See also Walker, "Shaping," e.g. ix.
80. Albert A. Schaal, "What must a FLOUR do?," *Good Housekeeping* (September 1950): 25; Albert A. Schaal, "What must a SHORTENING DO?," *Good Housekeeping* (July 1950): 25.; Renée Crucil, "Can these claims for fabrics *possibly* be true?," *Good Housekeeping* (August 1955): 6–8. On pseudoscientific terminology in women's periodical advertising see Nancy Tomes, *The Gospel of Germs: Men, Women, and the Microbe in American Life* (Cambridge: Harvard University Press, 1998), 248–49.

81. Historians analyzing this era point frequently to the equalizing of spousal relations, especially in the middle classes. See William Douglas, *Television Families: Is Something Wrong in Suburbia?* (Mahwah, NJ: Lawrence Erlbaum Associates, 2003), 79–80; and May, *Homeward Bound*, 146–53. May offers evidence as to the "professionalization" of parenting in this period. (Elaine Tyler May, *Homeward Bound*, 152; and *Barren in the Promised Land: Childless Americans and the Pursuit of Happiness* [New York: Basic Books, 1995], 132). This professionalization was promoted by popular medical advisors (e.g., Dr. Spock), reproductive technology, and the very entry of fathers into the parenting role in meaningful ways. (Elaine Tyler May, *Homeward Bound*, 149). By contrast, Mintz and Kellogg posit a more traditional (unbalanced/divided) structure for families during this period; the woman's main job, they argue, was still to serve her husband's professional, physical, and emotional needs. (Mintz and Kellogg, *Domestic Revolutions*, 186–87). Instead of a father newly involved in the lives of his children, the traditional situation of "father's absence forced the mother to assume the roles of both parents." (Mintz and Kellogg, *Domestic Revolutions*, 184).

82. Joe McCarthy, "Strike It Rich," *McCall's* (May 1952): 46ff.
83. Terry Morris, "The Amazing Case of the Eleven Orphans," *McCall's* (July 1952): 38ff.
84. Emily Martin, *Flexible Bodies: Tracking Immunity in American Culture from the Days of Polio to the Age of AIDS* (Boston: Beacon Press, 1994).
85. "What's Cooking with Barbecues?," *Good Housekeeping* (June 1950): 78–82.
86. She's Working *His* Way Through College," *McCall's* (March 1953): 32–35.
87. Eveylyn R. Zeek, "Mother Takes the Best Pictures," *McCall's* (February 1953): 20.
88. Ibid.

89. See also Walker, "Shaping," 147–48.

90. Dorothy Hartley, quoted in Elizabeth Sweeney Herbert, "This is How I Keep House," *McCall's* (July 1952) 68; Elizabeth Sweeney Herbert, "This is How I Keep House," *McCall's* (July 1952): 68.

91. Herbert, "This is How," 69. An even more emphatic statement on this issue—"There's Dust Under the Bed—So What!"—explicitly links fastidiousness with *bad* mothering and homemaking. A neighbor's "antiseptic housekeeping" (a condition ordinarily aimed for with every soap and scrubber on the market) is blamed by the easygoing author-persona for making visitors nervous, "trapp[ing her husband] in his spic-and-span home," and infecting her daughter with "the same kind of driven, compulsive orderliness." (Elizabeth Pope, "There's Dust Under the Bed—So What!," *McCall's* [June 1954]: 38.)

92. Herbert, "This is How," 70.

93. Ibid.

94. Ibid., 68.

95. Ibid.

96. Certainly the cultural significance of water images must have been a confused mix in the popular imagination. While the warm waters of pools and beaches during the polio months plainly indicated the danger of viral *infection*, the healthful properties of heated water—boiled for sterilization, FDR's own Warm Springs rehabilitation center, the steaming water used to heat strips of wool in the Kenny method of physical therapy—played large parts in the *treatment* stages of a post-acute polio attack. Thus one's feeling about the "health-giving" qualities of warm or cold water may have depended in large part on one's experience (personal or observed first hand) of being "pre" or "post" polio.

97. A recurring series in the *Journal*, Henry Safford's "Tell Me, Doctor," provides a striking example of misogynist abuse. Remarkable for its amateurish style and strongly slanted gender dynamics, the column presented advice in dramatized form—a nameless doctor welcomes a new patient each month and engages with her (and sometimes her husband) in long, circular debates about her "embarrassing" problems (pelvic tumor, tipped uterus, secret abortion). The two-dimensional female characters, complete with cardboard names like "Mrs. Black" and "Ms. White"—the patient from the first installment (February, 1950) was even named Jane Doe—feed the doctor questions in reliable straight-man fashion, providing the occasional "oh, I see," and tolerating the doctor's chiding condescension (the postabortion patient [December 1952] is roundly browbeaten) with grateful smiles. In one episode (September 1952), the woman is almost entirely absent, while the doctor and husband haggle over the former's qualifications; in another (October 1952), the doctor performs a pelvic examination as we read, cued as to where his hands are by his half-formed utterances about his patient's anatomy.

98. Charlotte Montgomery, "America's 11 Favorites," *Good Housekeeping* (July 1952): 42ff.

99. Charlotte Montgomery, "Gadgets and Accessories," *Good Housekeeping* (December 1952): 44ff.

100. Richard Frey, "What if *You* Caused an Accident?" Woman and the Family Security Series, *Good Housekeeping* (July 1952): 18ff.

101. Mollie Smart, "Smitty Gets His Tonsils Out," *McCall's* (January 1952): 10–12.

102. Toni Taylor, "Help Your Child GET WELL," *Redbook* (August 1952): 64ff.

103. One of Dad's most important "jobs," according to recent cultural analyses of families during this period, was to prevent the sissification of his sons at the hands of overbearing Mom. See Mintz and Kellogg, *Domestic Revolutions*, 190, and May, *Homeward Bound*, 146.

104. Josephine Kenyon, "The Convalescent Child," *Good Housekeeping* (February 1952): 28ff.

105. Leona Baumgartner, M.D., and Molly Castle, "Is Your Child Scared of the Doctor?," *McCall's* (October 1952): 130.

106. In fact, a piece for *McCall's* concedes that "Mother is the Best Cure for a Sick Child," emphasizing her capacity for providing "TLC" and even demonstrating the bed-changing skills necessary for patients who are so sick they cannot be moved (or cannot move) off the bed; however, as with the "Protecting Your Child from . . . Polio" piece described above (n. 40), this piece stands out for its brevity and singularity among so many other examples. (Aiken Welch and J. Leonard Moore, M.D., "Mother is the Best Cure for a Sick Child," *McCall's* [September 1951]: 104–7.)

2. "No Time for Tears"?

1. Charles H. Andrews, *No Time for Tears* (New York: Doubleday & Company, Inc., 1951), 27.

2. Ibid., 34.

3. Ibid., 84.

4. Ibid., 148.

5. See for instance Mairian Corker and Sally French, "Reclaiming Discourse in Disability Studies," in *Disability Discourse*, ed. Mairian Corker and Sally French (Buckingham: Open University Press, 1999), 1–11; Jenny Morris, *Pride Against Prejudice: Transforming Attitudes to Disabilities* (London: Women's Press, 1998); Margrit Shildrick, *Embodying the Monster: Encounters with the Vulnerable Self* (London: Sage, 2002); Margrit Shildrick and Janet Price, ed., *Vital Signs: Feminist Reconfigurations of the Bio/logical Body* (Edinburgh: Edinburgh University Press, 1998); and Carol Thomas. *Female Forms: Experiencing and Understanding Disability* (Buckingham: Open University Press, 1999).

6. See also Charles Mee, *A Nearly Normal Life: A Memoir* (Boston: Little, Brown, and Company, 1999), 90.

7. Virginia Lee Counterman Acosta, *Polio Tragedy of 1941* (Bloomington, IN: 1st Books, 1999), 8. Acosta's down-to-earth, unschooled narrative style is an example of a viewpoint rarely if ever entertained in print and therefore singularly valuable:

> In 1942 my mother took me to the fair in my wheel chair. There was no fair in 1941 because of polio. My mother said, "I think we will go see the livestock first." I said, "We always see the livestock last."
>
> We went to the barn where the cows were. As we went down to the end of the barn, there were a lot of people by this big cow. . . . There was my name and she had my name. Virginia Lee and she had a Blue Ribbon. The farmer and his wife and two sons said we hope you are not mad at us. We named our cow after you. I said, "I am so happy. I do not know what to say."
>
> . . . . Virginia the cow said, "Moo." I said to the cow that we will always be friends. Everyone laughed.

I became friends with the farmer and his family. I would go to see Virginia Lee the cow every weekend. Virginia Lee the cow was never put on the table. She passed away of old age. In 1956 when polio vaccine came, the cow passed away. (41–42)

8. Hugh Gregory Gallagher, *Black Bird Fly Away: Disabled in an Able-Bodied World* (Arlington, VA: Vandamere Press, 1998), 241.

9. G. Thomas Couser, *Recovering Bodies*, 5; see also 198.

10. See also Daniel J. Wilson, "Covenants of Work and Grace: Themes of Recovery and Redemption in Polio Narratives," *Literature and Medicine* 13, no.1 (1994): 23. Anne Hunsaker Hawkins notes that "As a genre, pathography is remarkable in that it seems to have emerged *ex nihilo*; book-length personal accounts of illness are uncommon before 1950 and rarely found before 1900." I infer from this observation that polio played a large part in inaugurating this popular genre. Hawkins, *Reconstructing Illness: Studies in Pathography* (West Lafayette, IN: Purdue University Press, [1993] 1999), 3.

11. Amy L. Fairchild, "The Polio Narratives: Dialogue with FDR," *Bulletin of the History of Medicine* 75 (2001): 488–534.

12. Rosemarie Garland Thomson, *Extraordinary Bodies: Figuring Physical Disability in American Culture and Literature* (New York: Columbia University Press, 1997).

13. David T. Mitchell and Sharon L. Snyder, *Narrative Prosthesis: Disability and the Dependencies of Discourse* (Ann Arbor: University of Michigan Press, 2000), 164.

14. Ibid., 169.

15. See for instance Colin Barnes, Mike Oliver, and Len Barton, eds. *Disability Studies Today* (Cambridge: Polity, 2002); Mairian Corker and Tom Shakespeare "Mapping the Terrain," in *Disability/Postmodernity: Embodying Disability Theory*, ed. Mairian Corker and Tom Shakespeare (London: Continuum, 2002), 1–17; Lennard J. Davis, *Bending Over Backwards: Disability, Dismodernism, and Other Difficult Positions* (New York: New York University Press, 2002) and *Enforcing Normalcy: Disability, Deafness, and the Body* (London: Verso, 1995); Tanya Titchkosky "Disability in the News: A Reconsideration of Reading," *Disability and Society* 20, no. 6 (2005): 655–68 and *Disability, Self, and Society* (Toronto: University of Toronto Press, 2003); Sally Tremaine, "On the Subject of Impairment," in *Disability/Postmodernity: Embodying Disability Theory* (London: Continuum, 2002), 32–47; and Susan Wendell, "Toward a Feminist Theory of Disability," in *The Disability Studies Reader*, ed. Lennard J. Davis (New York: Routledge, 1997), 260–78.

16. Liz Crow, "Including All of Our Lives: Renewing the Social Model of Disability," in *Exploring the Divide: Illness and Disability*, ed. Colin Barnes and Geof Mercer (Leeds: Disability Press, 1996), 60.

17. Davis, *Enforcing Normalcy*, 3–4.

18. For instance Carol Thomas (chapter 4) and Felicity Nussbaum, "Feminotopias: The Pleasures of 'Deformity' in Mid-Eighteenth-Century England," in *The Body and Physical Difference: Discourses of Disability*, ed. David T. Mitchell and Sharon L. Snyder (Ann Arbor: University of Michigan Press, 1997), 161–73.

19. Michael Oliver quoted in Shildrick and Price, *Vital Signs*, 228. In fact the divide is more mixed: David T. Mitchell and Sharon L. Snyder apply a social-model critique to older, outdated treatments of impaired literary figures but argue for the political efficacy of more recent, postmodern narratives, while Thomson sees effective representations of impairment in autobiographical texts by African American women authors, even though

she feels it is often misrepresented in mainstream literature. Mitchell and Snyder, *Narrative Prosthesis*; Thomson, *Extraordinary Bodies*, 11.

20. Corker and French, "Reclaiming Discourse," 4; see also Geyla Frank, *Venus On Wheels: Two Decades of Dialogue on Disability, Biography, and Being Female in America* (Berkeley: University of California Press, 2000), 56–57; Elizabeth C. Hamilton, "From Social Welfare to Civil Rights: The Representation of Disability in Twentieth-Century German Literature," in *The Body and Physical Difference: Discourses of Disability*, ed. David T. Mitchell and Sharon L. Snyder (Ann Arbor: University of Michigan Press, 1997), 223; and Shildrick and Price, *Vital Signs*.

21. See Howard Brody, *Stories of Sickness* (New Haven: Yale University Press, 1987), xiii; Tod Chambers and Kathryn Montgomery, "Plot: Framing Contingency and Choice in Bioethics," *Stories Matter: The Role of Narrative in Medical Ethics*, ed. Rita Charon and Martha Montello (New York: Routledge, 2002), 82; Rita Charon, "Time and Ethics," in *Stories Matter: The Role of Narrative in Medical Ethics*, ed. Rita Charon and Martha Montello (New York: Routledge, 2002), 61–62; and Hilda Lindemann Nelson, "Context: Backward, Sideways, Forward," in *Stories Matter: The Role of Narrative in Medical Ethics*, ed. Rita Charon and Martha Montello (New York: Routledge, 2002), 39–40.

22. Tod Chambers and Kathryn Montgomery, "Plot: Fraing Contingency and Choice in Bioethics," in *Stories Matter: The Role of Narrative in Medical Ethics*, ed. Rita Charon and Martha Montello (New York: Routledge, 2002, 81.

23. Cheryl Mattingly, *Healing Dramas and Clinical Plots: The Narrative Structure of Experience* (Cambridge: Cambridge University Press, 1998), 2.

24. Ibid., 16; see also Brody, *Stories*, 16–17 and Hawkins, "Introduction."

25. Cheryl Mattingly, "Emergent Narratives," in *Narrative and the Cultural Construction of Healing*, ed. Cheryl Mattingly and Linda C. Garro (Berkeley: University of California Press, 2001), 183–85.

26. Arthur Kleinman, M.D., *The Illness Narratives: Suffering, Healing, and the Human Condition* (New York: Basic Books, 1988), 48.

27. Arthur W. Frank, *The Wounded Storyteller: Body, Illness, and Ethics*. Chicago: University of Chicago Press, 1995, 22.

28. Ibid., 62.

29. Ibid., 63. See also Hawkins, *Reconstructing Illness*, 104–19 and G. Thomas Couser, "Signifying Bodies: Life Writing in Disability Studies," in *Disability Studies: Enabling the Humanities*, ed. Sharon L. Snyder, Brenda Jo Brueggeman, and Rosemarie Garland Thomson (New York: MLA, 2002), 109–17. Couser comfortably distinguishes "good books" and "the best personal accounts" (115) from among the plethora of recently published disability narratives. He observes that "autobiography deserves a prominent place in the rapidly developing discipline of disability studies" (109) but, heeding Davis's warning, acknowledges that it must be read critically, especially in the classroom.

30. Andrews, *No Time for Tears*, 16

31. Mary Grimley Mason, *Life Prints: A Memoir of Healing and Discovery* (New York: The Feminist Press at the City University of New York, 2000), 6.

32. Ibid., 38.

33. Ibid., 39.

34. Garrett Oppenheim with Gwen Oppenheim, *The Golden Handicap: A Spiritual Quest* (Virginia Beach, VA: A.R.E. Press, 1993), 3.

35. Ibid., 108.

36. Ibid., 109.

37. Robert C. Huse, *Getting There: Growing Up with Polio in the '30s* (Bloomington, IN: 1st Books, 2002), 19.

38. Ibid.

39. Ibid.

40. While treated only briefly, Charles L. Mee also describes his father's damaging, defeatist reaction to his illness and disability in his autobiography, *A Nearly Normal Life*. It is his father, Mee is sure, who called the Catholic priest to administer extreme unction during the boy's acute infection (22), a gesture that consigns him to death as he struggles to survive. Later, Mee is hurt by a picture his father carries with him, of his able-bodied son at football practice, a memento of "the last moment when my father felt uncomplicated pride in me. . . . I always took the fact that he carried that picture as a sign of his disappointment in me, and it filled me with rage" (171).

41. Anne Finger, *Elegy for a Disease: A Personal and Cultural History of Polio* (New York: St. Martin's Press, 2006), 168.

42. Daniel J. Wilson, "Crippled Manhood: Infantile Paralysis and the Construction of Masculinity," *Medical Humanities Review* 12, no. 2 (1998): 10.

43. Turnley Walker, *Rise Up and Walk* (New York: E.P. Dutton & Co., 1950), 82.

44. Wilson, "Crippled Manhood," 9.

45. Ibid., 22–23.

46. Kriegel quoted in Fairchild, "The Polio Narratives," 522.

47. Bentz Plagemann, *My Place to Stand* (New York: Farrar, Strauss, and Company, 1949), 11.

48. Ibid., 89.

49. Ibid., 155–59.

50. Leonard Kriegel, *Flying Solo: Reimagining Manhood, Courage, and Loss* (Boston: Beacon Press, 1998), 5.

51. Fairchild, "The Polio Narratives," 514.

52. Kriegel, *Flying Solo*, 139. The only text I have found to deal frankly with the subject of post-polio sexuality is Steve Carter's drama, *Nevis Mountain Dew* (1979). In the play, the revelation of the unorthodox sexual activities of Jared (who is in an iron lung) and his wife Billie catalyze the play's main crisis; in the scene immediately following, Jared pleads successfully with his family to end his life. While both the unchallenged perception of the couple's sexual activity as perversion and of Jared's death as cathartic and healing would be read critically from a disability studies standpoint, this text is unique in its graphic dealing with a quadriplegic protagonist's sexual circumstances, in its being a polio play that enjoyed at least one professional run—in New York in 1978—and in its being an African American-authored text, performed originally by an African American cast. Steve Carter, *Nevis Mountain Dew* (New York: Dramatists Play Services, Inc., [1978] 1979).

53. Meeting a woman whose polio-affected brother committed suicide, Kriegel in *Flying Solo* seeks to instill depth into their meandering dialogue with meaningless comments like, "'I'm not sure I understand,' I say. Only I understand all too well" (23) and "[Vietnam] wasn't just a war,' Harry says, frowning. I nod. 'But that doesn't stop me from wanting to believe it was.'" (25). Later, a man on crutches "who can go as far as the strength in his arms and the rage in his heart allow" (41) smacks of the melodramatic; throughout (e.g., 41), the poetical "beneath his shoulders" is preferred to the anatomical "armpit."

54. Kriegel, *Flying Solo*, 141.

55. Ibid., 32.
56. Ibid., 33.
57. Ibid., 39.
58. Ibid., 54.
59. Ibid., 44.
60. Gallagher, *Black Bird Fly Away*, 18.
61. Ibid., 39.
62. Ibid., 47.
63. A companion piece is the auto/biography by Diane Zemke Hawksford, *Polio: A Special Ride?* (1997) evidently written by herself but told in the first-person voice of her stated "Subject": "My Brother — Ron Zemke." Interesting reversals result from the fact that Ron was a small boy when polio happened to him, making "his own" story the product of other's memories, as will be the case of Kathryn Black, discussed later in this chapter. In one striking passage, "I [a 17-month-old boy] of course have no memory of that day, but my sister has vivid memories of the difficulties my parents encountered gaining my release [from the polio hospital]" (11). The book's cover photo is of a merry-go-round, emblematic of Hawksford's subtitle, "A Special Ride"; on the back, Zemke smiles affably in the upper photo while in the lower one, Hawksford's *back is to the camera* as she rides away on a merry-go-round horse. Diane Zemke Hawksford, *Polio: A Special Ride?* (Minnotonka, MN: The Diagnostic Center of Learning Patterns, 1997).
64. Anne Buck Walters and Jim Marugg, *Beyond Endurance* (New York: Harper and Brothers, 1954), 4. Elsewhere, Marugg imagines himself the target of the House Un-American Activities Committee. Singular in its effort to analyze the connection between the era's twin terrors — polio and communism (or, in Marugg's case, false accusation of communist infiltration) — Marugg later hallucinates a sign on the iron lung mirror of another patient — "Marugg is a Communist" — that causes the medical staff to ignore and mistreat him (25). See also Kenneth Kingery, who recreates the derangement of acute infection by recalling that "Live Indians and wild cornflakes poured shrieking and singing from a nearby radio." Kenneth Kingery, *As I Live and Breathe* (New York: Grosset and Dunlap, 1966), 25.
65. Walters and Marugg, *Beyond Endurance*, 6.
66. Ibid., 33.
67. Fairchild, "The Polio Narratives," 528.
68. Eleanor Chappell, *On the Shoulders of Giants: The Bea Wright Story* (Philadelphia: Chilton Company, 1960), 17–18.
69. Ibid., 24.
70. Ibid., 23–24.
71. Ibid., 19.
72. Ibid., 23.
73. Ibid., 25.
74. Ibid., 22.
75. Ibid., 47–48.
76. Hayes, Helen, "Foreword." *On the Shoulders of Giants: The Bea Wright Story* by Eleanor Chappell (Philadelphia: Chilton Company, 1960), vii.
77. Mason, 71.
78. Ibid., 151.
79. Ibid., 102.

80. Fairchild, "The Polio Narratives," 529–30.

81. Paralleling Mason's story of dysfunctional marriages among the academic elite is Judy Hoit's working-class account of the heartache caused by her deadbeat husband, *My World has Access Now*. As reticent regarding her polio impairment as is Mason, Hoit is abandoned by her alcoholic husband just before the birth of their first child, without a word from Hoit as to how this affects her. Following his absence, the couple simply "got back together" (23), while later Arnold gets "help for his alcoholism" (25). The Hoits later divorce, decide to reunite, and part for good at Arnold's behest: "I was informed by Arnold, in front of his [substance abuse] counselor, that he would not be coming home. He said he didn't love me anymore and wanted to be alone. I was crushed. I remember crying in front of the counselor and being embarrassed" (33). Judy Hoit, *My World Has Access Now* (Iowa City: Access Now, 1992).

82. Noreen Lidunska, *My Polio Past* (Chicago: Pellegrini and Cudahy, 1947), 30.

83. Ibid., 39.

84. Fairchild, "The Polio Narratives," 505.

85. Jane Boyle Needham, as told to Rosemary Taylor, *Looking Up* (New York: G. Putman & Sons, 1959), 189–90.

86. Kathryn Black, *In the Shadow of Polio: A Personal and Social History* (Reading, MA: Addison-Wesley, 1996), 17.

87. Ibid., 17–18.

88. Ibid., 123.

89. Ibid., 59.

90. Mark O'Brien with Gillian Kendall, *How I Became a Human Being: A Disabled Man's Quest for Independence* (Madison: University of Wisconsin Press, 2003), 15.

91. Ibid., 258–59.

92. Louis Sternberg and Dorothy Sternberg with Monica Dickens, *View from the Seesaw* (New York: Dodd, Mead & Company, 1986), 101–2.

93. Ibid., 18.

94. Ibid., 19.

95. Ibid.

96. Ibid.

97. Ibid., 41.

98. Ibid.

99. Ibid.

100. Ibid., 50.

101. Ibid., 95, 147–48.

102. Larry Alexander, *The Iron Cradle* (New York: Cromwell, 1954), 203.

103. Kingery, *As I Live and Breathe*, 112–13 and passim.

104. Ibid., 80.

105. Ibid., 116.

106. Ibid., 104.

107. Ibid., 130.

108. Ibid., 129–30.

109. Ibid., 162–63.

110. See also Arthur Frank, *The Wounded Storyteller*, 138–42, who reads the term much less ironically than I do, and Hawkins, *Reconstructing Illness*, 4.

111. See also Wilson, "A Crippling Fear: Experiencing Polio in the Era of FDR," *Bulletin of the History of Medicine* 72 (1998): 467.

112. See also Anne Borsay, "History, Power, and Identity," in *Disability Studies Today*, ed. Colin Barnes, Mike Oliver, and Len Barton (Cambridge: Polity, 2002), 115.

113. I therefore dissent from Linda C. Garro's argument that "Bartlett, who first talked of remembering in terms of reconstruction, claimed that in 'a world of constantly changing environment, literal recall is extraordinarily unimportant.'" Linda C. Garro, "Cultural Knowledge as Resource in Illness Narratives: Remembering Through Accounts of Illness," in *Narrative and Cultural Construction of Illness and Healing*, ed. Cheryl Mattingly and Linda C. Garro (Berkeley: University of California Press, 2000), 71. By contrast, Arthur Frank describes an "ethic of recollection" whereby "displaying one's past to others requires taking responsibility for what was done" (132). Also Marc Shell works insightfully with the tension between memory and forgetting in *Polio and Its Aftermath*. He observes that, as we have forgotten polio texts (and experiences) since the vaccine, so these texts themselves often sent the recurring message—to their polio protagonists and readers—that "it's best to not look back" (51).

114. Arnold R. Beisser, *Flying Without Wings: Personal Reflections on Being Disabled* (New York: Doubleday, 1989), 12.

115. Mee, *A Nearly Normal Life*, 12.

116. Ibid., 121.

117. Ibid., 120.

118. Ibid., 213.

119. Ibid., 164.

120. Black, *In the Shadow of Polio*, 199.

121. Ibid., 51.

122. Ibid., 262.

123. Ibid., 189.

124. Ibid., 249.

125. Ibid., 56.

126. Mee, *A Nearly Normal Life*, 69.

127. See Marilynne Rogers, "Of Iron Lungs and Wheelchairs / Marilynne Rogers," *Polio's Legacy: An Oral History*, ed. Edmund J. Sass with George Gottfried and Anthony Sorem (Lanham: University Press of America, 1996), 57. See also Larry Alexander, *The Iron Cradle* (New York: Cromwell, 1984) and Lynne M. Dunphy, "'The Steel Cocoon': Tales of Nurses and Patients of the Iron Lung, 1929–1955," *Nursing History Review* 9 (2001): 3–33. Respirator patients have described panic upon reintroduction to unassisted breathing, seeking out the safety of the iron lung during times of stress or overnight.

128. Hawkins, *Reconstructing Illness*, 115.

129. Wilfrid Sheed, *In Love with Daylight: A Memoir of Recovery* (Pleasantville, NY: Akadine Press, [1995] 1999), 19.

130. Black, *In the Shadow of Polio*, 179.

131. Kriegel quoted in Black, 178.

132. Lauro S. Halstead, M.D., and Gunnar Grimby, M.D., PhD., *Post-Polio Syndrome* (Philadelphia: Hanley and Belfus, Inc., 1995), 201.

133. Halstead quoted in Black, 178.

134. Gallagher, *Black Bird Fly Away*, 177.

135. Ibid., 246.

136. Ibid., 178.

137. Ibid., 34–35.
138. Lorenzo Wilson Milam, *The Cripple Liberation Front Marching Band Blues* (San Diego: Mho & Mho Works, 1984), 67.
139. Ibid., 93.
140. Ibid., 108; see also Needham, *Looking Up*, 51.
141. This is the title of a 1963 polio memoir by British authors Paul Bates and John Pellow.
142. Milam, *The Cripple Liberation*, 103.
143. Interestingly, Gallagher is mentioned in an anecdote in Milam's memoir, when both men, graduate students together, ogle a healthy young man in a gym locker, combining lust and envy in an amorphous longing to both *have* and *be* the able-bodied male form (111). Gallagher's own story plays tenuously with the prospect of sexual ambivalence or closeted gay identity, and various of his obituaries—he died of cancer in 2004—indicate gay activism, membership in the gay/lesbian/transgender organization for Catholics known as Dignity, and a male partner among his survivors. Yet Gallagher never came out in print; his writing thus leaves open the question as to whether self-closeting complicates the original picture of physical impairment, depression, and social/sexual isolation.
144. Milam, *The Cripple Liberation*, 69.
145. Kriegel, *Flying Solo*, 48.
146. Ibid., 54.
147. Ibid., 55.
148. Beisser, *Flying without Wings*, 18.
149. Mee, *A Nearly Normal Life*, 32.
150. Ibid., 18.
151. Ibid., 19.
152. I recognize that critique of mind/body dualism is an essential component of much theorizing in literature-medicine studies; Arthur Frank's comment eloquently represents the problem: "Only a caricature Cartesianism would imagine a head compartmentalized away from disease, talking about the sick body beneath it" (2). While Beisser and Mee both work toward integration of them/selves in their lives and writing, we must acknowledge that the iron lung occupation and below-the-neck paralysis characteristic of severe polio infections lend themselves perfectly to figurative mind/body severance, and both writers make powerful use of the image.
153. Beisser, 133.
154. Ibid., 143.
155. Ibid., 29.
156. As noted above the philosophers discussed here (Mee and Beisser) are both men; see Couser, *Recovering Bodies*, 185.
157. Mee, *A Nearly Normal Life*, 33.
158. Ibid., 23.
159. Beisser, *Flying without Wings*, 156.
160. Ibid., 133.
161. Arthur Frank, *The Wounded Storyteller*, 115.
162. Sternberg, *View from the Seasaw*, 207.
163. Ibid., 91–92.
164. Thomas, *Female Forms*, 68.

3. "Crippled by History"

1. In fact many Americans continue to suffer from polio-related impairments acquired in the mid-twentieth century, and post-polio syndrome has begun to affect many more among the mildly or unimpaired as they enter advanced age. Jerrold Hirsch has spoken effectively against the tendency to think of polio as having ended with the vaccination. Jerrold Hirsch, "History and a Story of Polio: Using and Abusing Oral History Narratives," *Disability Studies Quarterly* 18, no. 4 (1998): 65. I fully share this sentiment but am phrasing here the mainstream perception of polio's pastness and analyzing novels that disseminate this perception. As aware as I am that polio is still very much a part of the American present (and future, especially the future of disability rights), I recognize also the value of *historical awareness* in all contexts and am mining these texts for their historical insight.

2. James Baldwin, "Sonny's Blues," 1957, *The Norton Introduction to Literature*, ed. Jerome Beaty, et al. (New York: W.W. Norton & Company, 2002), 41–64.

3. Shell, *Polio and Its Aftermath*, 7.

4. Ibid., 23.

5. Ibid., 207, 218.

6. Ibid., 10.

7. An exception is Elsie Oakes Barber's *The Trembling Years* (New York: MacMillan Company, [1949] 1959), a novel about polio with nonfiction origins, being based on Barber's personal experience with the disease. It is remarkable for its close adherence to the polio memoir format, which follows the protagonist, Kathy Storm, who got polio at seventeen, as Barber did, from illness onset through satisfying recovery; all but one of the novels to be considered in this discussion (Stegner's) take their polio protagonists well beyond the initial polio experience, while the vast majority set polio illness so far in the protagonist's past that it is barely treated at all. The *New York Times* critiqued Barber's overly idyllic love story and slick style but congratulated its "vividness and emotional intensity" (Ann Schakne, "Stricken Adolescence," review of *The Trembling Years*, *New York Times Book Review* [April 17, 1949], 18). Despite the mixed review, and its low quality with respect to plot, character, and style, the novel seems to have filled what was perceived even then as a significant cultural gap, having had thirteen printings by 1959. (My thanks to Gordon Hutner for calling this novel to my attention.) Similarly, Ann L. McLaughlin's much more recent *Lightning in July* (Santa Barbara: John Daniel, 1989) stays focused on the illness and recovery of the story's protagonists, who come down with polio the same day, are sent to the same hospital to recuperate, and eventually fall in love. Like Barber's, this story began as a memoir in the 1950s, which McLaughlin had trouble selling at that time, so retooled as polio fiction several decades later to satisfy market interest. ("Summer of '55," *Book World* [February 18, 1990], 15.)

8. As Jane S. Smith aptly notes, the National Foundation for Infantile Paralysis was a "wonderful show" (*Patenting the Sun*, 80), and the publicists, journalists, and fundraisers who worked for the organization "peddled polio the same way they could have sold cars or corsets or annuities" (81). Neither a government agency nor a private charity, it blended individual commitment and collective support. So great was the response to the call to split polio's devastating cost among every family able to contribute that the Foundation was as dependable (in fact, in the 1930s, much more dependable) than the bank, the insurance company, or the federal government (see also Shell, 181–86).

9. See Ellen Feldman, *Lucy* (New York: W.W. Norton & Company, 2003) and Rhoda Lerman, *Eleanor* (New York: Holt, Rinehart, and Winston, 1979). Although both authors did historical research to substantiate their novelizations of the Roosevelts' personal lives, each is primarily a romance novel that emphasizes relationships, sanctioned and illicit, while inserting history in somewhat obvious ways and downplaying polio overall.

10. Wallace Stegner, *Crossing to Safety* (New York: Random House, 1987), 180.

11. I am indebted to Brad Isaacs for helping me to this observation.

12. David T. Mitchell and Sharon L. Snyder, eds., "Introduction: Disability Studies and the Double Bind of Representation," in *The Body and Physical Difference: Discourses of Disability* (Ann Arbor: University of Michigan Press, 1997), 6.

13. Tom Shakespeare, "Art and Lies?: Representation and Disability on Film," in *Disability Discourse*, ed. Mairian Corker and Sally French, 164 (Buckingham: Open University Press, 1999).

14. Or any sort of ending at all. In Julie Harris's *The Longest Winter* (New York: St. Martin's Press, 1995), the protagonist's sister Meg has polio, but she is kept off-stage until the novel's final pages. Following her brother's long absence among Inuit natives following a plane crash, the reunion with Meg accompanies the novel's transition from the ahistorical, romanticized Alaskan environment to the mainland and the passage of time as marked by historic events (specifically World War II). "Lack[ing] imagination" in their childhood, she is sour of personality and underwhelmed by her brother's return. If polio accounts for her bad attitude, it also spoils the dramatic payoff of the siblings' reunion, furthering our sense of polio's reduced, perfunctory role in the story.

15. Martin Norden, *The Cinema of Isolation: A History of Physical Disability in the Movies* (New Brunswick, NJ: Rutgers University Press, 1994), 1.

16. Thomson, *Extraordinary Bodies*, 9.

17. Davis, *Enforcing Normalcy*, 49.

18. Ibid., 41.

19. Thomson, *Extraordinary Bodies*, 10.

20. David T. Mitchell, "Narrative Prosthesis and the Materiality of Metaphor," *Disability Studies: Enabling the Humanities*, ed. Sharon L. Snyder, Brenda Jo Brueggeman, and Rosemarie Garland Thomson (New York: Modern Language Association, 2002), 15–30.

21. Davis, *Enforcing Normalcy* (chap. 6); Kriegel, "The Wolf in the Pit at the Zoo," *Social Policy* 13, no.2 (1982): 16–23; and Sanjeev Kumor Uprety, "Disability and Postcoloniality in Salman Rushdie's *Midnight's Children* and Third-World Novels," in *The Disability Studies Reader*, ed. Lennard J. Davis (New York: Routledge, 1997), 366–81.

22. Howard Brody, *Stories of Sickness* (New Haven: Yale University Press, 1987), xiii.

23. Thomson, *Extraordinary Bodies*, 9, and Deborah Kent, "In Search of a Heroine: Images of Women with Disabilities in Fiction and Drama," in *Women with Disabilities: Essays in Psychology, Culture, and Politics*, ed. Michelle Fine and Adrienne Asche (Philadelphia: Temple University Press, 1988), 94.

24. Mitchell, "Narrative Prosthesis," 23.

25. Ibid.

26. See esp. Adrienne Asch and Michelle Fine, "Nurturance, Sexuality, and Women with Disabilities: The Example of Women and Literature," in *The Disability Studies Reader*, ed. Lennard J. Davis, 241–59 (New York: Routledge, 1997); Amy L. Fairchild;

Thomson, *Extraordinary Bodies*; Susan Wendell, "Toward a Feminist Theory of Disability," in *The Disability Studies Reader*, ed. Lennard J. Davis (New York: Routledge, 1997), 260–78; and Wilson, "Crippled Manhood."

27. Daniel Wilson, *Living with Polio: The Epidemic and Its Survivors* (Chicago: University of Chicago Press, 2005), 208–16.

28. In an interesting counterargument, Shell isolates the repeated theme of the "premature ending of childhood" in several of the polio nonfictions he studies (30).

29. James Carroll, *Secret Father* (Boston: Houghton Mifflin, 2003), 231.

30. In the hospital, Brian's circle of tough-talking pals are wonderfully brought to life:

> "What happens if you have to take a crap?" asked Bernie, from his list of topical questions.
> "They got pots and pans for that. You lose your taste for it after awhile." Fact. He was brimming with constipation. But did they really want to hear about that? . . . . Stranded between jollity and reverence, his friends hardly knew where to turn.

Wilfrid Sheed, *People Will Always Be Kind* (New York: Farrar, Straus, and Giroux, 1973), 19–20.

When Brian's especially terrified friend Hennessy in fact succumbs to polio the following summer, Brian and his family express sorrow to the friend who brings the news, then break into horrible, heartfelt celebration when he has gone: "And the three old hypocrites made a long face over it. A while after that, Kevin put on some records, including his collection of Irish jigs, and he and Beatrice did a couple of steps, the way they used to do them at the Irish Reeling Society before Brian had ever been thought of" (123).

31. Sheed, *People Will Always Be Kind*, 171.
32. Ibid., 236.
33. Ibid., 368.
34. Ibid., 369.
35. Ibid., 363.
36. Ibid., 299.
37. Anne Finger, *Bone Truth* (Minneapolis: Coffee House Press, 1994), 63.
38. Ibid., 91.
39. Ibid., 14.
40. Ibid., 176.
41. Ana Castillo, *Peel My Love Like an Onion* (New York: Doubleday, 1999), 94.
42. Ibid., 153.
43. Ibid., 123–24.
44. Related to Castillo's less than total engagement with the issue of disability is her unfortunately typical treatment of an AIDS-affected character in her story. Paul K. Longmore has critiqued authors who depict disabled characters who themselves turn away from able-bodied friends, thus deserving the isolation they end up with. Longmore, "Screening Stereotypes: Images of Disabled People," *Social Policy* 16, no. 1 (1985), 36. We read of Carmen's failing relationship to Virgil: "Once he started getting sick all the time, we didn't see each other anymore. I called him a few times with no return calls, then silence. I only hear about him now through his sister." Castillo, *Peel My Love*, 112.
45. Castillo, *Peel My Love*, 101.

46. David Leavitt, *Equal Affections* (New York: Weidenfeld & Nicolson, 1989), 147.
47. Ibid., 148.
48. Ibid., 185.
49. Ibid., 223.
50. Stegner, *Crossing to Safety*, 195.
51. Ibid., 167.
52. Ibid., 170.
53. Ibid., 212.
54. Ibid., 167.
55. Ibid., 220.
56. Ibid., 241.
57. Howard Owen, *Answers to Lucky* (New York: Harper Collins Publishers, 1996), 72.
58. Ibid., 212.
59. Stegner, *Crossing to Safety*, 180.
60. Rona Jaffe, *The Road Taken* (New York: Penguin Putnam, 2000), 178–79.
61. Dorothy Uhnak, *The Ryer Avenue Story* (New York: St. Martin's Press, 1993), 316.
62. Ibid., 145.
63. Ibid., 145–46.
64. Jaffe, *The Road Taken*, 250.
65. Ibid., 363.
66. Ibid., 324.
67. Frank Deford, *An American Summer* (Naperville, IL: Sourcebooks, Inc., 2002), 227.
68. Nancy Mairs, "Sex and Death and the Crippled Body: A Meditation," *Disability Studies: Enabling the Humanities*, ed. Sharon L. Snyder, Brenda Jo Brueggeman, and Rosemarie Garland Thomson (New York: Modern Language Association, 2002), 162.
69. Wendell, "Toward a Feminist Theory," 268.
70. See also Martha Stoddard Holmes, "The Twin Structure: Disabled Women in Victorian Courtship Plots," in *Disability Studies: Enabling the Humanities*, ed. Sharon L. Snyder, Brenda Jo Brueggemann, and Rosemarie Garland Thomson (New York: MLA, 2002), 222–33.
71. Deford, *An American Summer*, 171.
72. Ibid., 74.
73. Ibid., 48
74. Ibid., 83.
75. Ibid., 61.
76. Ibid., 119.
77. Ibid., 141.
78. Ibid., 192.
79. Ibid., 58.
80. Ibid., 2, ellipsis in original.
81. "Skee-Ball is a game where you roll a little wooden ball down a short bowling ally-type thing" (66).
82. Ibid., 102.
83. Ibid., 45.
84. Ibid., 181.

85. For instance, ibid., 19, 103, 220.
86. Pat Cunningham Devoto, *My Last Days as Roy Rogers* (New York: Warner Books, 1999), ix.
87. Ibid.
88. Ibid., 264.
89. Ibid., 277.
90. Ibid., 200.
91. Ibid., 309.
92. Ibid., 29.
93. Ibid., 47.
94. Ibid., 73.
95. Ibid., 167.
96. Ibid., 291.
97. Thomson, *Extraordinary Bodies*, 105.
98. Davis, *Bending Over Backwards*, 7.
99. Devoto, *My Last Days*, 355.
100. We might read the novel's faulty racial politics in either case: despite Davis's productive analogizing of race, class, and disability oppression, the white middle class in America often regards its racial and classed others as *more* physically adept than they—faster, stronger, more athletic, better skilled in manual labor—and cultivates a fair-skinned, leisured, pampered, even immobilized ideal in opposition. While it is possible that Maudie May died on her arduous journey to far-flung rehab facilities because it is her culturally inscribed role to do so, it is more likely that she survived in spite of these travails because her hearty, impervious peasant-stock origins suit her especially, almost comfortably or naturally, to hardship and deprivation. Naomi Rogers has studied the racial politics of polio rehabilitation, describing a history of segregated services, when services were available at all. While by the early 1950s polio's victimization of young black children "helped to make polio a more palatable issue [than syphilis] for civil rights activism," it is significant that Maudie May is not especially young, small, feminine, or sweet – that is, that she is no one's idea of a polio poster child. Rogers, "Race and the Politics of Polio," *American Journal of Public Health* 97, no. 5 (2007), 793.
101. Devoto, *My Last Days*, 356.
102. Paul K. Longmore, "Screening Stereotypes: Images of Disabled People," *Social Policy* 16, no. 1 (1985): 31–37, 36.
103. Tony Earley, *Jim the Boy* (New York: Little, Brown and Company, 2000), 225.
104. Ibid.
105. Ibid., 227.
106. Michael Köepf, *The Fisherman's Son* (New York: Broadway Books, 1998), 211.
107. Ibid., 130.
108. Ibid., 211.
109. Ibid.
110. Ibid., 232.
111. Michael Chabon, *The Amazing Adventures of Kavalier and Clay* (New York: Random House, 2000), 255.
112. Robert McRuer, "Compulsory Able-Bodiedness and Queer/Disabled Existence," in *Disability Studies: Enabling the Humanities*, ed. Sharon L. Snyder, Brenda Jo Brueggeman, and Rosemarie Garland Thomson (New York: Modern Language Association, 2002), 94.

113. After his lover Tracy Bacon leaves for a career in Hollywood, Sammy never attempts to find another partner, as the conventions of the time push him (and the unmarried, pregnant Rosa) into a sham marriage. Likewise, a fellow comic writer blames Sammy's mid-life business failures on his propensity for

> "*sidekicks*. It's like an obsession with him. . . . He takes over a character, first thing he does, no matter what, he gives the guy a little pal. . . . All of a sudden the Stallion's hanging around with this kid, what was his name? Buck something."
> "Buck Naked."
> "Buckskin. The kid gunslinger. . . . " (481)

114. Chabon, *Amazing Adventures*, 145.
115. Carroll, *Secret Father*, 197.
116. Ibid., 221.
117. Ibid., 120
118. Ibid., 110.
119. Ibid., 74.
120. Ibid., 288.
121. Ibid., 225.
122. Ibid., 247.
123. Ibid., 336.
124. James Patterson, *Cradle and All* (New York: Little, Brown and Company, 2000), 14.
125. Ibid., 45.
126. Ibid., 268.
127. Ibid., 280.
128. Dean Coonts, *Cuba* (New York: St. Martin's Paperbacks, 1999), 214.
129. Ibid., 120.
130. Ibid., 14–15, 231.
131. For instance, Kent, "In Search of a Heroine,"; Mitchell and Snyder, "Introduction" and *Narrative Prosthesis*; and Thomson, *Extraordinary Bodies*.

4. "Heads, You Win!"

1. See Dick Goodwin, "History and Philosophy of the Independent Living Movement." *Impact On Line: Independent Living Philosophy and History*, February–April, 1991, http://www.impactcil.org/general_info/written/il_phil/ilphilosophy.html;> and Joan Headley, "Independent Living: The Role of Gini Laurie," *Post-Polio Health International*, October 1997, http://www.post-polio.org/hist-gini.html, February 24, 2004.
2. Sue Williams and Gini Laurie, letter to Kathryn D. Goodwin, Director of Bureau of Public Assistance, Department of Health, Education, and Welfare (May 11, 1961), 1. March of Dimes Archive, Public Relations Records collection, Box 17, File: "Rehabilitation Gazette, 1959–1970."
3. Ibid.
4. Harlan Lane, "Constructions of Deafness," *The Disability Studies Reader*, ed. Lennard J. Davis (New York: Routledge, 1997), 155.
5. Leonard J. Davis, *Enforcing Normalcy: Disability, Deafness, and the Body* (London: Verso, 1995), 75.

6. Benedict Anderson, *Imagined Communities: Reflections on the Origin and Spread of Nationalism* (London: Verso, 1983), 47; Davis, *Enforcing Normalcy*, 75.

7. Leonard J. Davis, *Bending over Backwards: Disability, Dismodernism, and Other Difficult Positions* (New York: New York University Press, 2002), 102.

8. All issues of Warm Springs' newsletters, including the *Polio Chronicle*, the *Daily Crutch*, *The Crutch*, and the *Wheelchair Review*, in addition to all issues of the *Toomey j. Gazette*, the *Rehabilitation Gazette*, *Post-Polio Health*, and *Ventilator-Assisted Living* cited in this study were accessed at the Roosevelt Warm Springs Institute for Rehabilitation, Research Library, Founders Hall, Warm Springs, Georgia.

9. Roosevelt's foundations (both the Warm Springs Foundation and the National Foundation, the March of Dimes) commingled many sectors—politics, business, science, enormous amounts of private donations—suggesting significant conflicts of interest: were the foundations primarily self-serving—encouraging a cure for Roosevelt's own affliction and earning himself if not dollars then the votes necessary to return to the White House four times? Could celebrities endorsing Roosevelt's March of Dimes help but endorse his presidency as well? Were the only celebrities marching for dimes left-wing democrats, or was it political suicide for a movie star to miss the polio bandwagon, no matter how he or she voted? Was there ever the implication that right-wing foes of Roosevelt seeking Foundation support acted hypocritically in their requests, or did the polio crisis supersede the bitterly divided politics of this period, uniting adversaries in the shared goal of helping and receiving help? Historian David Oshinsky observes that in fact the March of Dimes's early fundraising events, the annual presidential Birthday Balls, were run very much along party lines and that many Washington conservatives "refused to support a charity so intimately connected to a man they despised." Oshinsky, *Polio: An American Story* (new York: Oxford University Press, 2005), 52.

10. Davis, *Enforcing Normalcy*, 98.

11. See Oshinsky, *Polio*, 36–37.

12. Marc Shell, Polio and Its Aftermath: *The Paralysis of Culture* (Cambridge, MA: Harvard University Press, 2005), 118.

13. Davis, *Enforcing Normalcy*, 85.

14. My searches at the Tuskegee archive have failed to turn up a newsletter-type publication for African Americans recovering from polio at that institution in the postwar period. Tuskegee was informally designated as the "negro Warm Springs" and evidently served its segregated population well. See Rogers, "Race and the Politics of Polio."

15. *The Crutch* (November 15, 1937), 2.

16. Ibid., 1.

17. Ibid., 3A.

18. Ibid., 2. Interestingly, the *Crutch*'s conservative precursor, the *Chronicle*, referred to prejudices against those with polio marrying able-bodied girls as "tommyrot" (May 1933).

19. *The Crutch* (November 15, 1937), 3

20. *The Crutch* (November 22, 1938), 8.

21. *Wheelchair Review* (September 9, 1951), 6.

22. *Wheelchair Review* (August 12, 1951), 5.

23. *Wheelchair Review* (June 25, 1955), 11.

24. *Wheelchair Review* (September 27, 1951), 1.

25. *Wheelchair Review* (August 12, 1951), 5.

26. Ibid.

27. *Wheelchair Review* (July 27, 1951), 10.

28. Grant Heilman and Marjorie Heilman, "Polio Parents, Inc," *The Woman* with *Woman's Digest* (July 1950), 49. While the Swarthmore group seems to have been especially active, polio parents' clubs sprang up across the country and worked in unofficial tandem with their local March of Dimes chapters. The MOD grew nervous, not surprisingly, when various of these amateur-run groups began spreading medical misinformation, though for the most part they were social clubs providing networks of emotional support, not information centers or fundraisers as were the March of Dimes chapter offices. The newsletter of the Swarthmore group kept members abreast of "club activities," and Grant and Marjorie Heilman observe helpfully, despite their unfortunate choice of terms, that "[t]o shut-ins, mail can be the most important thing in the world" (48).

29. *Wheelchair Review* (August 12, 1951), 7.

30. See for instance, Asch and Fine, "Nurturance, Sexuality, and Women with Disabilities"; Holmes, "The Twin Structure"; Mairs, "Sex and Death and the Crippled Body"; Thomson, "Feminist Theory, the Body, and the Disabled Figure," in *The Disability Studies Reader*, ed. Lennard J. Davis (New York: Routledge, 1997), 279–92; and Wendell, "Toward a Feminist Theory of Disability."

31. Corker and French, "Reclaiming Discourse in Disability Studies," 7.

32. *Wheelchair Review* (February 23, 1952), 5.

33. The marked similarity between Warm Spring's *Wheelchair Review* and the monthly newsletter of southern California's polio/respirator center at Rancho Los Amigos, *The Weakly Breather*, suggests that the editors of both publications were regular, inspired readers of each other's work. Not only is the *Breather*'s focus on personal information, trivia, gossip, in-jokes, and an unflinching interest in the physical aspects of polio living laid out in slap-dash, dynamic style nearly identical to that of the *Review*; archives for both centers indicate near-identical careers of style changes over the years. As in Warm Springs, Rancho's newsletter was more employee- than patient-focused in its early formats, enjoyed a thematic and stylistic heyday in the mid to late '50s (in its *Weakly Breather* incarnation), and overproduced itself with respect to cover art and contents pages in the 1960s and 1970s, losing its vital poliocentric and somacentric focus as it did.

34. Reading copies of the Northwest Respirator Center's *Vital Capacitator*, in the course of her memoir of her mother's tragic involvement with respiratory polio, Kathryn Black feels off-put and deceived by the upbeat tone of pieces written by her mother and others, as it conflicts with moods of sorrow and depression that prevailed in the ward as remembered by caretakers interviewed by Black: "Living with other severely handicapped people, Mother also had plenty of reminders of the fragility of her existence. Often a patient choked or a breathing machine failed. What next? Who next? . . . . Despite the cheerfulness of 'The Vital Capacitator' reports, . . . fears and anxieties circulated in the respirator room at Harborview." Black, *In the Shadow of Polio*, 144. Indeed, it is likely that the atmosphere at polio rehab centers crossed the spectrum from upbeat and collegial as at the well-funded Warm Springs to grim and futile as at lower-quality facilities in parts of the country that cared less about or had less to spend upon its polio-impaired citizens.

35. Despite the suggestive title, the *Post*, sponsored by the Charlottetown Orthopedic Centre on Prince Edward Island, reported on all of the Centre's activities and provided very few articles about polio per se. Its two "personals" columns, entitled "Scene: Here / Overheard at the Centre" and "Kiddie Kwotes," indicate an interest in patients' personal

doings, similar to the intensely focused reporting of the *Crutch* and *Review*, but in fact ascribe to actual patients canned jokes and well-worn aphorisms. Another quarterly publication, Ireland's Infantile Paralysis Fellowship's *Polio Journal*, seemed also designed for a "general interest" audience; its advertising, fiction, humor, columns, and feature stories rarely mentioned polio.

36. All issues of *Accent on Living*, *Polio Living*, and the Charlottetown *Polio Post* cited in this study were accessed at the National Library of Medicine, Bethesda, Maryland.

37. Davis, *Enforcing Normalcy*, 82.

38. "Should the Handicapped Consider Marriage?" *Accent on Living* (Summer 1960). 14–16; Duncan A. Holbert, M.D., "Sex and the Disabled," *Toomey j. Gazette* 10 (1967): 14–15.

39. For instance, *Accent on Living* (Spring 1970): 32–34.

40. William R. Scales's, "Battle of the Bathroom," *Accent on Living* (Winter 1969): 28–31.

41. *Toomey j. Gazette* (August 1958), 2.

42. In the Summer 1959 issue, the editors inform their readership that they have "coined a new word to describe us — Respos" — to substitute for the lengthy and cumbersome "respiratory polios" that might have seemed the more polite term. Meanwhile, even calling someone a "polio" strikes the modern ear as demeaning and inappropriate, no better than the term it in-part supplanted, "paral," used by the writers of the *Polio Chronicle* back in Warm Springs's early days: in August 1932, "There was a paral from the Bronx ["pronounced "Bronnix"] / Who wasn't so good on harmonx; / But she married a guy / Whose income was high —/ Now her braces are studded with onx."

43. *Toomey j. Gazette* (Winter 1958–59): 2.

44. *Toomey j. Gazette* (Spring 1959): n.p.

45. Editor's introduction to "Hobbies" by Duncan A. Holbert, M.D., *Rehabilitation Gazette* (1974): 40.

46. Holbert, "Sex and the Disabled," 15.

47. Editor's note to Elbridge S. Rector, "Warning to Others: A Letter to Ponder," *Toomey j. Gazette* 6, no. 1 (1963): 41.

48. Joan Headley, personal interview, July 30, 2007.

49. *Post-Polio Health* 11, no. 2 (Spring 1995): 8.

50. *Post-Polio Health* 11, no. 1 (1995): 6–7.

51. Anderson, *Imagined Communities*, 42. Significantly, the questions of human suffering Anderson sees religion as once having answered are all disability-related: "Why was I born blind? Why is my best friend paralysed? Why is my daughter retarded?" (18).

Conclusion

1. Martin Norden, *The Cinema of Isolation: A History of Physical Disability in the Movies* (New Brunswick, NJ: Rutgers University Press, 1994) 3; see also Robert Bogdan et al, "The Disabled: Media's Monsters," *Social Policy* 13, no. 2 (1982): 32–35; Lauri E. Klobas, "Introduction," in *Disability Drama in Television and Film* (Jefferson, NC: McFarland & Company, 1988), xi–xviii; and Paul K. Longmore, "Screening Stereotypes: Images of Disabled People," *Social Policy* 16, no. 1 (1985): 31–37.

2. See for instance Hugh Gregory Gallagher, *FDR's Splendid Deception* (Arlington, VA: Vandamere Press, 1994).

3. Norden, *Cinema*, 1.

4. Interestingly, both Lawrence and Kenny were Australian natives who moved on to success in America and world fame. "Marjorie Lawrence used the treatment developed by Sister Elizabeth Kenny when the performer contracted poliomyelitis in 1941." "Australian Women—Biographical Entry," http://www.womenaustralia.info/biogs/IMP0157b.htm.

5. Yet as Lauri E. Klobas observes, "access is rarely discussed in dramas" involving wheelchair users (114), and this film indeed avoids details regarding how Lawrence overcame the logistical difficulties of her tour.

6. Norden, *Cinema*, 3, 4.

7. In addition to Greer Garson's 1961 nomination for her supporting role as Eleanor in *Sunrise at Campobello*, Eleanor Parker and Rosiland Russell were both nominated for their leading roles in their respective polio films. In addition, *Interrupted Melody* was nominated for best costume design in a color film and won the award for Best Story and Screenplay. *Sunrise* did win five Tony Awards.

Works Cited

Acosta, Virginia Lee Counterman. *Polio Tragedy of 1941*. Bloomington, IN: 1st Books, 1999.

Alexander, Larry. *The Iron Cradle*. New York: Cromwell, 1954.

Anderson, Benedict. *Imagined Communities: Reflections on the Origin and Spread of Nationalism*. London: Verso, 1983.

Andrews, Charles H. *No Time for Tears*. New York: Doubleday & Company, Inc., 1951.

Asche, Adrienne, and Michelle Fine. "Nurturance, Sexuality, and Women with Disabilities: The Example of Women and Literature." In *The Disability Studies Reader*, edited by Lennard J. Davis, 241–59. New York: Routledge, 1997.

"Australian Women-Biographical Entry." Online. <http://www.womenaustralia.info/biogs/IMP0157b.htm>

Baldwin, James. "Sonny's Blues." In *The Norton Introduction to Literature*, edited by Jerome Beaty, et al, 41–64. New York: W.W. Norton & Company, [1957] 2002.

Barber, Elsie Oakes. *The Trembling Years*. New York: MacMillan Company, [1949] 1959.

Barnes, Colin, Mike Oliver, and Len Barton, eds. *Disability Studies Today*. Cambridge: Polity, 2002.

Beisser, Arnold R. *Flying Without Wings: Personal Reflections on Being Disabled*. New York: Doubleday, 1989.

Belknap, E. Clinton. *Nebraska and the Fight Against Polio, 1944–1965: An Album Compilation*. Lincoln, NE: Self-published, 1982.

Berger, John. *Ways of Seeing*. London: British Broadcasting Corporation and Penguin Books, [1972] 1977.

Black, Kathryn. *In the Shadow of Polio: A Personal and Social History*. Reading, MA: Addison-Wesley, 1996.

Bogdan, Robert et al. "The Disabled: Media's Monsters." *Social Policy* 13, no. 2 (Fall 1982): 32–35.

Borsay, Anne. "History, Power, and Identity." In *Disability Studies Today*, edited by Colin Barnes, Mike Oliver, and Len Barton, 98–119. Cambridge: Polity, 2002.

Brody, Howard. *Stories of Sickness*. New Haven: Yale University Press, 1987.

Carroll, James. *Secret Father*. Boston: Houghton Mifflin, 2003.

Carter, Steve. *Nevis Mountain Dew*. New York: Dramatists Play Services, Inc., [1978] 1979.

Castillo, Ana. *Peel My Love Like an Onion*. New York: Doubleday, 1999.

Chabon, Michael. *The Amazing Adventures of Kavalier and Clay*. New York: Random House, 2000.

Chambers, Tod, and Kathryn Montgomery. "Plot: Framing Contingency and Choice in Bioethics." *Stories Matter: The Role of Narrative in Medical Ethics*, edited by Rita Charon and Martha Montello, 77–84. New York: Routledge, 2002.

Chappell, Eleanor. *On the Shoulders of Giants: The Bea Wright Story*. Philadelphia: Chilton Company, 1960.

Charon, Rita. "Time and Ethics." In *Stories Matter: The Role of Narrative in Medical Ethics*, edited by Rita Charon and Martha Montello, 59–68. New York: Routledge, 2002.

Coonts, Stephen. *Cuba*. New York: St. Martin's Paperbacks, 1999.

Corker, Mairian and Sally French, eds, *Disability Discourse*. Buckingham: Open University Press, 1999.

———. "Reclaiming Discourse in Disability Studies." In *Disability Discourse*, edited by Mairian Corker and Sally French, 1–11. Buckingham: Open University Press, 1999.

——— and Tom Shakespeare, ed. "Mapping the Terrain." In *Disability/Postmodernity: Embodying Disability Theory*, 1–17. London: Continuum, 2002.

Couser, G. Thomas. *Recovering Bodies: Illness, Disability, and Life Writing*. Introduction Nancy Mairs. Madison: University of Wisconsin Press, 1997.

———. "Signifying Bodies: Life Writing in Disability Studies." In *Disability Studies: Enabling the Humanities*, edited by Sharon L. Snyder, Brenda Jo Brueggeman, and Rosemarie Garland Thomson, 109–17. New York: MLA, 2002.

Crow, Liz. "Including All of Our Lives: Renewing the Social Model of Disability." *Exploring the Divide: Illness and Disability*, edited by Colin Barnes and Geof Mercer, 55–73. Leeds: Disability Press, 1996.

The Crutch. National Patients' Committee of the Georgia Warm Springs Foundation. Warm Springs, GA: 1951(?)–1955(?).

The Daily Crutch. National Patients' Committee of the Georgia Warm Springs Foundation. Warm Springs, GA: early 1950s.

Davis, Lennard J. *Bending Over Backwards: Disability, Dismodernism, and Other Difficult Positions*. New York: New York University Press, 2002.

———. *Enforcing Normalcy: Disability, Deafness, and the Body*. London: Verso, 1995.

Deford, Frank. *An American Summer*. Naperville, IL: Sourcebooks, Inc., 2002.

Devoto, Pat Cunningham. *My Last Days as Roy Rogers*. New York: Warner Books, 1999.

Douglas, William. *Television Families: Is Something Wrong in Suburbia?* Mahwah, NJ: Lawrence Erlbaum Associates, 2003.

Dunphy, Lynne M. "'The Steel Cocoon': Tales of Nurses and Patients of the Iron Lung, 1929–1955." *Nursing History Review* 9 (2001): 3–33.

Earley, Tony. *Jim the Boy*. New York: Little, Brown and Company, 2000.

Editor's introduction to "Hobbies" by Duncan A. Holbert, M.D. *Rehabilitation Gazette* (1974): 40.

Endres, Kathleen L., and Therese L. Lueck, ed. *Women's Periodicals in the United States: Consumer Magazines*. Westport, CT: Greenwood Press, 1995.

Fairchild, Amy L. "The Polio Narratives: Dialogue with FDR." *Bulletin of the History of Medicine* 75 (2001): 488–534.

Feldman, Ellen. *Lucy*. New York: W.W. Norton & Company, 2003.

Ferguson, Marjorie. *Forever Feminine: Women's Magazines and the Cult of Femininity*. London: Heinemann, 1983.

Finger, Anne. *Bone Truth*. Minneapolis: Coffee House Press, 1994.

———. *Elegy for a Disease: A Personal and Cultural History of Polio*. New York: St. Martin's Press, 2006.

Frank, Arthur W. *The Wounded Storyteller: Body, Illness, and Ethics*. Chicago: University of Chicago Press, 1995.

Frank, Geyla. *Venus On Wheels: Two Decades of Dialogue on Disability, Biography, and Being Female in America*. Berkeley: University of California Press, 2000.

Gallagher, Hugh Gregory. *Black Bird Fly Away: Disabled in an Able-Bodied World*. Arlington, VA: Vandamere Press, 1998.

———. *FDR's Splendid Deception*. Arlington, VA: Vandamere Press, 1994.

Garro, Linda C. "Cultural Knowledge as Resource in Illness Narratives: Remembering Through Accounts of Illness." In *Narrative and Cultural Construction of Illness and Healing*, edited by Cheryl Mattingly and Linda C. Garro, 70–87. Berkeley: University of California Press, 2000.

Goodwin, Dick. "History and Philosophy of the Independent Living Movement." In *Impact On Line: Independent Living Philosophy and History*. February–April, 1991. <http://www.impactcil.org/general_info/written/il_phil/ilphilosophy.html>

Gould, Tony. *A Summer Plague: Polio and Its Survivors*. New Haven: Yale University Press, 1995.

The Gulper's Gazette. Buffalo Polio Respiratory Center Edited by Diane Bacon. Buffalo, NY: 1955(?).

Hall, Robert F. *Through the Storm: A Polio Story*. St. Cloud, MN: North Start Press of St. Cloud, 1990.

Halstead, M.D., Lauro S., and Gunnar Grimby, M.D., PhD. *Post-Polio Syndrome*. Philadelphia: Hanley and Belfus, Inc., 1995.

Hamilton, Elizabeth C. "From Social Welfare to Civil Rights: The Representation of Disability in Twentieth-Century German Literature." In *The Body and Physical Difference: Discourses of Disability*, edited by David T. Mitchell and Sharon L. Snyder, 223–39. Ann Arbor: University of Michigan Press, 1997.

Harris, Julie. *The Longest Winter*. New York: St. Martin's Press, 1995.

"Harvey W. Wiley: Pioneer Consumer Activist," *Good Housekeeping* February 1990. 145–46.

Hawkins, Anne Hunsaker. *Reconstructing Illness: Studies in Pathography*. 1993. 2nd ed. West Lafayette, IN: Purdue University Press, 1999.

Hawksford, Diane Zemke. *Polio: A Special Ride?* Minnotonka, MN: The Diagnostic Center of Learning Patterns, 1997.

Hayes, Helen. "Foreword." In *On the Shoulders of Giants: The Bea Wright Story* by Eleanor Chappell, vii–viii. Philadelphia: Chilton Company, 1960.

Headley, Joan L. "Independent Living: The Role of Gini Laurie." *Post-Polio Health International*. October, 1997. <http://www.post-polio.org/hist-gini.html> February 24, 2004.

———. Personal interview. July 30, 2007.

Heilman, Grant, and Marjorie Heilman. "Polio Parents, Inc." *The Woman* with *Woman's Digest* (July 1950): 46–49.

Hirsch, Jerrold. "History and a Story of Polio: Using and Abusing Oral History Narratives." *Disability Studies Quarterly* 18, no. 4 (Fall 1998): 264–66. Rpt. as "Disability

History and a Story of Polio: Using and Abusing Oral History Narratives." *Rehabilitation Gazette* 39, no. 2 (1999). February 29, 2003. <http://www.post-polio.org/gini/rg39-2.html#disa>

Hoit, Judy. *My World Has Access Now*. Iowa City: Access Now, 1992.

Holbert, Duncan A. "Sex and the Disabled." *Toomey j. Gazette* 10 (1967): 14–15.

Holmes, Martha Stoddard. "The Twin Structure: Disabled Women in Victorian Courtship Plots." In *Disability Studies: Enabling the Humanities*, edited by Sharon L. Snyder, Brenda J. Brueggemann, and Rosemarie Garland Thomson, 222–33. New York: MLA, 2002.

Huse, Robert C. *Getting There: Growing Up with Polio in the '30s*. Bloomington, IN: 1st Books, 2002.

Interrupted Melody. Directed by Curtis Bernhardt. MGM, 1955.

Jaffe, Rona. *The Road Taken*. New York: Penguin Putnam, 2000.

Kent, Deborah. "In Search of a Heroine: Images of Women with Disabilities in Fiction and Drama." In *Women with Disabilities: Essays in Psychology, Culture, and Politics*, edited by Michelle Fine and Adrienne Asche, 90–110. Philadelphia: Temple University Press, 1988.

Kingery, Kenneth. *As I Live and Breathe*. New York: Grosset and Dunlap, 1966.

Kleinman, M.D., Arthur. *The Illness Narratives: Suffering, Healing, and the Human Condition*. New York: Basic Books, 1988.

Klobas, Lauri E. *Disability Drama in Television and Film*. Jefferson, NC: McFarland & Company, 1988.

Kluger, Jeffrey. *Splendid Solution: Jonas Salk and the Conquest of Polio*. New York: G.P. Putnam's Sons, 2005.

Köepf, Michael. *The Fisherman's Son*. New York: Broadway Books, 1998.

Kriegel, Leonard. *Flying Solo: Reimagining Manhood, Courage, and Loss*. Boston: Beacon Press, 1998.

———. "The Wolf in the Pit at the Zoo." *Social Policy* 13, no. 2 (1982): 16–23.

Lane, Harlan. "Constructions of Deafness." In *The Disability Studies Reader*, edited by Lennard J. Davis, 153–71 New York: Routledge, 1997.

Leave Her to Heaven. Directed by John M. Stahl. Twentieth Century Fox, 1946.

Leavitt, David. *Equal Affections*. New York: Weidenfeld & Nicolson, 1989.

Lerman, Rhoda. *Eleanor*. New York: Holt, Rinehart, and Winston, 1979.

Lidunska, Noreen. *My Polio Past*. Chicago: Pellegrini and Cudahy, 1947.

Longmore, Paul K. "Screening Stereotypes: Images of Disabled People." *Social Policy* 16, no. 1 (1985): 31–37.

Mairs, Nancy. "Sex and Death and the Crippled Body: A Meditation." In *Disability Studies: Enabling the Humanities*, edited by Sharon L. Snyder, Brenda Jo Brueggeman, and Rosemarie Garland Thomson, 156–70. New York: Modern Language Association, 2002.

Martin, Emily. *Flexible Bodies: Tracking Immunity in American Culture from the Days of Polio to the Age of AIDS*. Boston: Beacon Press, 1994.

Mason, Mary Grimley. *Life Prints: A Memoir of Healing and Discovery*. New York: The Feminist Press at the City University of New York, 2000.

Mattingly, Cheryl. *Healing Dramas and Clinical Plots: The Narrative Structure of Experience*. Cambridge: Cambridge University Press, 1998.

———. "Emergent Narratives." In *Narrative and the Cultural Construction of Healing*, edited by Cheryl Mattingly and Linda C. Garro, 181–211. Berkeley: University of California Press, 2001.

May, Elaine Tyler. *Barren in the Promised Land: Childless Americans and the Pursuit of Happiness*. New York: Basic Books, 1995.

———. *Homeward Bound: American Families in the Cold War Era*. New York: Basic Books, 1988.

McLaughlin, Ann L. *Lightning in July*. Santa Barbara: John Daniel, 1989.

McRuer, Robert. "Compulsory Able-Bodiedness and Queer/Disabled Existence." In *Disability Studies: Enabling the Humanities*, edited by Sharon L. Snyder, Brenda Jo Brueggeman, and Rosemarie Garland Thomson, 88–99. New York: Modern Language Association, 2002.

Mee, Charles L. *A Nearly Normal Life: A Memoir*. Boston: Little, Brown, and Company, 1999.

Milam, Lorenzo Wilson. *The Cripple Liberation Front Marching Band Blues*. San Diego: Mho & Mho Works, 1984.

Mintz, Steven, and Susan Kellogg. *Domestic Revolutions: A Social History of American Family Life*. New York: Free Press, 1988.

Mitchell, David T. "Narrative Prosthesis and the Materiality of Metaphor." In *Disability Studies: Enabling the Humanities*, edited by Sharon L. Snyder, Brenda Jo Brueggeman, and Rosemarie Garland Thomson, 15–30. New York: Modern Language Association, 2002.

Mitchell, David T., and Sharon L. Snyder, eds. "Introduction: Disability Studies and the Double Bind of Representation." In *The Body and Physical Difference: Discourses of Disability*, 1–31. Ann Arbor: University of Michigan Press, 1997.

———. *Narrative Prosthesis: Disability and the Dependencies of Discourse*. Ann Arbor: University of Michigan Press, 2000.

Morris, Jenny. *Pride Against Prejudice: Transforming Attitudes to Disabilities*. London: Women's Press, 1998.

Mott, Frank Luther. *A History of American Magazines*. 5 vols. Cambridge, MA: Harvard University Press, 1938–68.

Needham, Jane Boyle, as told to Rosemary Taylor. *Looking Up*. New York: G. Putman & Sons, 1959.

Nelson, Hilde Lindemann. "Context: Backward, Sideways, Forward." In *Stories Matter: The Role of Narrative in Medical Ethics*, edited by Rita Charon and Martha Montello, 39–47. New York: Routledge, 2002.

Norden, Martin. *The Cinema of Isolation: A History of Physical Disability in the Movies*. New Brunswick, NJ: Rutgers University Press, 1994.

Nussbaum, Felicity. "Feminotopias: The Pleasures of 'Deformity' in Mid-Eighteenth-Century England." In *The Body and Physical Difference: Discourses of Disability*, edited by David T. Mitchell and Sharon L. Snyder, 161–73. Ann Arbor: University of Michigan Press, 1997.

O'Brien, Mark with Gillian Kendall. *How I Became a Human Being: A Disabled Man's Quest for Independence*. Madison: University of Wisconsin Press, 2003.

Oppenheim, Garrett with Gwen Oppenheim. *The Golden Handicap: A Spiritual Quest*. Virginia Beach, VA: A.R.E. Press, 1993.

Oshinsky, David M. *Polio: An American Story*. New York: Oxford University Press, 2005.

Owen, Howard. *Answers to Lucky*. New York: Harper Collins Publishers, 1996.

Patterson, James. *Cradle and All*. New York: Little, Brown and Company, 2000.

Plagemann, Bentz. *My Place to Stand*. New York: Farrar, Strauss, and Company, 1949.

The Polio Chronicle. National Patients' Committee of the Georgia Warm Springs Foundation. Warm Springs, GA: 193?–1937(?).

Polio Journal. Infantile Paralysis Fellowship (Ireland). Dublin: 1953–1968(?).

Polio Living (later *Accent on Living* 1958–2001). Edited by Raymond Cheever. Bloomington, IL: 1956–1958.

The Polio Post. Prince Edward Island Orthopedic Center. Charlottetown, PEI: 1953(?)–19?.

Rector, Elbridge S. "Warning to Others: A Letter to Ponder." *Toomey j. Gazette* 6, no. 1 (1963): 41.

Reed, David. *The Popular Magazine in Britain and the United States, 1880–1960*. London: British Library, 1997.

Rogers, Marilynne. "Of Iron Lungs and Wheelchairs / Marilynne Rogers." In *Polio's Legacy: An Oral History*, edited by Edmund J. Sass with George Gottfried and Anthony Sorem, 54–61. Lanham: UP of America, 1996.

Rogers, Naomi. *Dirt and Disease: Polio Before FDR*. Rutgers: Rutgers University Press, 1992.

———. "Race and the Politics of Polio." *American Journal of Public Health* 97, no. 5 (2007): 784–95.

Sass, Edmund J. with George Gottfried and Anthony Sorem. *Polio's Legacy: An Oral History*. Lanham: University Press of America, 1996.

Scales, William R. "Battle of the Bathroom." *Accent on Living* (Winter, 1969): 29–31.

Schakne, Ann. "Stricken Adolescence." Review of *The Trembling Years*. *New York Times Book Review* (April 17, 1949): 18.

Shakespeare, Tom. "Art and Lies?: Representation and Disability on Film." In *Disability Discourse*, edited by Mairian Corker and Sally French. Buckingham: Open University Press, 1999. 164–72.

Sheed, Wilfrid. *In Love with Daylight: A Memoir of Recovery*. 1995. Pleasantville, NY: Akadine Press, 1999.

———. *People Will Always Be Kind*. New York: Farrar, Straus, and Giroux, 1973.

Shell, Marc. *Polio and its Aftermath: The Paralysis of Culture*. Cambridge, MA: Harvard University Press, 2005.

Shildrick, Margrit. *Embodying the Monster: Encounters with the Vulnerable Self*. London: Sage, 2002.

Shildrick, Margrit, and Janet Price, eds. *Vital Signs: Feminist Reconfigurations of the Bio/logical Body*. Edinburgh: Edinburgh University Press, 1998.

Silver, M.D., Julie K. *Post-Polio Syndrome: A Guide for Survivors and Their Families*. New Haven: Yale University Press, 2001.

Sister Kenny. Directed by Dudley Nichols. RKO Radio, 1946.

Smith, Jane S. *Patenting the Sun: Polio and the Salk Vaccine*. New York: Anchor/Doubleday, 1990.

SpeciaLiving. Edited by Betty Garee. Bloomington, IL: 2001–present.

The Spokesman. Edited by Charles Lyser. San Mateo, CA: Bay Counties Post-Polio Association, 1950s(?).

Stegner, Wallace. *Crossing to Safety*. New York: Random House, 1987.

Sternberg, Louis, and Dorothy Sternberg, with Monica Dickens. *View from the Seesaw*. New York: Dodd, Mead & Company, 1986.

"Summer of '55." *Book World*. February 18, 1990: 15.

Sunrise at Campobello. Directed by Vincent J. Donehue. Warner Brothers, 1960.

Thomas, Carol. *Female Forms: Experiencing and Understanding Disability*. Buckingham: Open University Press, 1999.

Thomson, Rosemarie Garland. *Extraordinary Bodies: Figuring Physical Disability in American Culture and Literature*. New York: Columbia University Press, 1997.

– – –. "Feminist Theory, the Body, and the Disabled Figure." In *The Disability Studies Reader*, edited by Lennard J. Davis, 279–92. New York: Routledge, 1997.

Titchkosky, Tanya. "Disability in the News: A Reconsideration of Reading." *Disability and Society* 20, no. 6 (2005): 655–68.

– – –. *Disability, Self, and Society*. Toronto: University of Toronto Press, 2003.

Tomes, Nancy. *The Gospel of Germs: Men, Women, and the Microbe in American Life*. Cambridge: Harvard University Press, 1998.

Toomeyville Jr. Gazette (later *Toomey j. Gazette* 1959–1970 and *Rehabilitation Gazette* 1970–2003). Edited by Sue Williams and Gini Laurie. Cleveland, OH: Cleveland Metropolitan General Hospital/Toomey Pavilion, 1958–1959.

Tremaine, Shelley. "On the Subject of Impairment." In *Disability/Postmodernity: Embodying Disability Theory*, edited by Mairian Corker and Tom Shakespeare, 32–47. London: Continuum, 2002.

Uhnak, Dorothy. *The Ryer Avenue Story*. New York: St. Martin's Press, 1993.

Uprety, Sanjeev Kumor. "Disability and Postcoloniality in Salman Rushdie's *Midnight's Children* and Third-World Novels." In *The Disability Studies Reader*, edited by Lennard J. Davis, 366–81. New York: Routledge, 1997.

Walker, Nancy A. *Shaping Our Mothers' World: American Women's Magazines*. Jackson: University of Mississippi Press, 2000.

Walker, Turnley. *Rise Up and Walk*. New York: E.P. Dutton & Co., 1950.

– – –. *Roosevelt and the Warm Springs Story*. New York: A.A. Wyn, 1953.

Walters, Anne Buck and Jim Marugg. *Beyond Endurance*. New York: Harper and Brothers, 1954.

The Weakly Breather. Edited by G. Barnett, M.D. Downey, CA: Rancho Los Amigos Hospital, 1952–1959.

Wendell, Susan. "Toward a Feminist Theory of Disability." In *The Disability Studies Reader*, edited by Lennard J. Davis, 260–78. New York: Routledge, 1997.

Williams, Sue and Gini Laurie. Letter to Kathryn D. Goodwin. May 11, 1961. March of Dimes Public Relations Records, Box 17, File: "Rehabilitation Gazette, 1959–1970."

Williams, Susanne. Personal iInterview. January 21, 2004.

Wilson, Daniel J. "Covenants of Work and Grace: Themes of Recovery and Redemption in Polio Narratives." *Literature and Medicine* 13, no. 1 (Spring 1994): 22–41.

———. "A Crippling Fear: Experiencing Polio in the Era of FDR." *Bulletin of the History of Medicine* 72 (1998): 464–95.

———. "Crippled Manhood: Infantile Paralysis and the Construction of Masculinity." *Medical Humanities Review* 12, no. 2 (1998): 9–28.

———. *Living with Polio: The Epidemic and Its Survivors*. Chicago: University of Chicago Press, 2005.

Magazine Citations from Chapter 1

From Good Housekeeping

Crucil, Renée. "Can these claims for fabrics *possibly* be true?" (August 1955): 6–8.
Davis, Maxine. "First Complete Handbook on Infantile Paralysis" (August 1950): 56ff.
Frey, Richard. "Your Child's Camp and POLIO" (May 1950): 54ff.
———. "What if *You* Caused an Accident?" Woman and the Family Security Series (July 1952): 18ff.
"The Girls in the Front Office." Town Hall series (July 1952): 14–15.
Kenyon, Josephine H. "The Convalescent Child" (February 1952): 28ff.
McCarthy, Joe. "Frothingham" (July 1950): 60ff.
Montgomery, Charlotte. "America's 11 Favorites" (July 1952): 4ff.
———. "Gadgets and Accessories" (December 1952): 44ff.
Schaal, Albert A. "What must a FLOUR do?" (September 1950): 25.
———. "What must a SHORTENING DO?" (July 1950): 25.
Porter, Sylvia F. "What to do in a PANIC" (June 1950): 54ff.
"What's Cooking with Barbecues?" (June 1950): 78–82.

From Ladies Home Journal

Briggs, Peter. "Conquering a New Disease" (May 1955): 133.
Bundesen, Dr. Norman H. "Protecting Your Child From Polio" (July 1950): 133–34.
Hickey, Margaret, ed. "Have We Won the Fight Against Polio?" (December 1954): 25ff.
"If Polio Strikes My Home" (June 1952): 86.
Killilea, Marie. "She Lived a Miracle" (August 1952): 36ff.
Safford, M.D., Henry B. "Tell Me Doctor" series.
Stuart, Neal G. "Year of Conquest over Polio" (October 1956): 187ff.

From McCall's

Baumgartner, M.D., Leona and Molly Castle. "Is Your Child Scared of the Doctor?" (October 1952): 130.
"A Boy's Summer" (July 1954): 26–29.
Charles, Felix. "I'm Proud of My Lies" (January 1952): 89.

Clark, Margaret. "Polio is Being Defeated" (January 1953): 48ff.
Gordon, Arthur. "The Doctor Speaks Out" (February 1953): 17ff.
Hayes, Helen. "I Learned to Live Through Heartbreak" (July 1952): 34ff.
Herbert, Elizabeth Sweeney. "This is How I Keep House" (July 1952): 68ff.
Holliday, Kate. "The Disease that Imitates POLIO" (August 1952): 42ff.
Kaufman, Suzanne. "Summer Bachelor" (September 1950): 28ff.
Landon, Dr. John Fitch. "The Questions You Ask the Doctor about Summer Problems" (July 1953): 95.
McCarthy, Joe. "Strike It Rich" (May 1952): 46ff.
McDermott, William F. "The House that Kindness Built" (August 1953): 36ff.
McNeill, Kay, as told to Isabella Taves. "10 Million Women are in Love with my Husband" (July 1951): 32ff.
Miller, Laura Owen. "Dangerous Summer" (May 1952): 38ff.
Miller, Maggie. "The Fair-Weather Kind" (February 1952): 46ff.
Morris, Terry. "The Amazing Case of the Eleven Orphans" (July 1952): 38ff.
"Mother, Beware" (October 1952): 22.
Pope, Elizabeth. "There's Dust Under the Bed—So What!" (June 1954): 38ff.
"She's Working *His* Way Through College" (March 1953): 32–35.
Smart, Mollie. "Smitty Gets His Tonsils Out" (January 1952): 10–12.
Taves, Isabella. "Jane Froman: Courage Unlimited" (May 1952): 30ff.
Van Riper, M.D., Hart. "What You Should Know about Polio Prevention" (March 1954): 136–37.
Welch, Aiken and J. Leonard Moore, M.D. "Mother is the Best Cure for a Sick Child" (September 1951): 104–7.
Zeek, Evelyn R. "Mother Takes the Best Pictures" (February 1953): 20–22.

From Redbook

Black, Irma Simonton. "Don't Fence Me In!" (November 1952): 73.
———. "Let the Kids Cook!" (October 1952): 93.
Fontaine, André. "The Town that Fought For Its Kids" (July 1950): 46ff.
Grissom, Grace I., as told to Jhan and June Robbins. "I Can Do Anything but Walk" (October 1955): 43ff.
Henry, Vera. "Free as a Gull" (April 1952): 32ff.
Miller, Floyd. "Camp is *Good* For 'Em!" (May 1952): 52ff.
"Polio Pledge" (September 1952): 86.
Smollar, M.D., Leo. "It Won't Kill You!" (May 1952): 21ff.
Taylor, Toni. "Help Your Child GET WELL" (August 1952): 64ff.
White, Lionel. "The Girl Who Never Gave Up" (June 1952): 46ff.

Index

ableism, examples of, 12, 17, 18, 23–24; in film, 171, 174, 175, 200 n. 44
Accent on Living (magazine), 138, 148, 153–158, 165, 168
Acosta, Virginia Lee Counterman, 190–91, n. 7
AIDS, 109, 113, 200 n. 44
Alexander, Larry, 78
All Iowa Reads program, 167
Amazing Adventures of Kavalier and Clay, The (novel), 99, 125–28, 203 n. 113
American Summer, An (novel), 112, 116–19
Andrews, Charles H., 22, 51, 52, 74
Answers to Lucky (novel), 110–12
Atlas, Charles, 127
atomic bomb, 44, 49, 102, 118, 184 n.3

Baldwin, James, 97, 101
Barber, Elsie Oakes, 198 n. 7
Bates, Paul, 197 n. 141
Beisser, Arnold, 84, 85, 90, 90–93, 95, 197 nn. 152 and 156
Belknap, E. Clinton, 153
Bellamy, Ralph, 173
Berle, Milton, 33
Berlin Wall, 101, 126, 129–30
Bernhardt, Curtis, 170
Better Homes and Gardens, 184 n. 3
Beyond Endurance (memoir), 67, 194 n. 64
birthday balls, 16
Black Bird Fly Away (memoir), 66
Black, Irma Simonton, 186 n. 41
Black, Kathryn, 72, 74–75, 80–86, 94–95, 194 n. 63, 205 n. 34
Blood, Virginia, 29

Bone Truth (novel), 62, 105–6
Breakfast Club, The (radio program), 32
Breathing Lessons (film), 76
Buffalo Polio Respiratory Center, 152
Bundesen, Norman, MD, 186 n. 40

Campobello Island, 15
Carroll, James, 23, 125, 126, 128, 131
Carter, Steve, 193 n. 52
Castillo, Ana, 106–108, 112, 200 n. 44
Chabon, Michael, 99, 125, 131
chaos narrative, 88
Chappell, Eleanor, 68, 71, 74, 81–82, 84, 85, 94–95
childhood: in women's magazines, 35–43, 187 n. 47; in memoirs, 200 n. 28; in novels, 99, 101–3
communism, 44, 49, 105, 184 n.3, 194 n. 64
Coonts, Stephen, 131–33
Coxsackie virus, 33, 34
Cradle and All (novel), 131–32
Crossing to Safety (novel), 99, 108, 110
Crutch (newsletter), 141–45, 152, 205–6 n. 35
Cuba (novel), 131–133

Daily Crutch (newsletter), 152
Deaf culture, 137, 138
"Dear Abby," 145
"Dear Bonnie," 156, 165
Deford, Frank, 112, 113, 116–19, 121–22, 126
denial: in polio texts, 14, 22, 53–54, 56, 62, 85–94; in polio survivors, 53, 85

219

depression, 30, 53, 55, 71, 83, 85–87, 94
Depression Era, 28, 61, 113
Devoto, Pat Cunningham, 112, 113, 119, 126
Disability Rag (newsletter), 167
Disability Rights Education and Defense Fund, 168
disability studies, 18–19, 57–58, 99–101, 102
Disability Studies-Temple U (blog), 167
Disability World (electronic magazine), 167
Donehue, Vincent J., 170
Ducas, Dorothy, 29

Earley, Jim, 123, 125
Eleanor (novel), 199 n. 9
Elegy for a Disease (memoir), 62
Equal Affections (novel), 108–10

fathers: in polio memoirs, 59–63, 77, 193 n. 40; in polio novels, 103, 111–12, 129
Feldman, Ellen, 199 n. 9
feminism: in disability studies, 18, 54, 57–58; in postwar women's magazines, 43–47
Finger, Anne, 62, 105
Fisherman's Son, The (novel), 123, 124–25
Flying Solo (memoir), 65
Flying Without Wings (memoir), 84
Ford, Glenn, 173
Froman, Jane, 33
Freud, Sigmund, 52, 127

Gallagher, Hugh Gregory, 66, 68, 86–88, 92–93, 197 n. 143
Galliard, Tim, 34
Garson, Greer, 173, 207 n. 7
gender, 19, 21, 27, 188 n. 81, 190 n. 103; in polio memoirs, 51–80; in polio novels, 113, 114–15, 123
Gimp Parade, The (blog), 167
Good Housekeeping, 27, 30, 35, 36, 44, 48, 184 nn. 3 and 6
"good story, the" 59, 192 n. 29
Guillaume-Barré Syndrome, 183 n. 11

Gulper's Gazette (newsletter), 152

Hall, Robert F., 11, 84
Halstead, Lauro S., MD, 86–87
Harris, Julie, 199 n. 14
Hartley, Dorothy, 46–47
Hawksford, Diane Zemke, 194 n. 63
Hayes, Helen, 32, 69, 70, 184 n. 15
Headley, Joan, 166
healthboards.com (online discussion group), 167
Hitler, Adolph, 112, 128
Hobby, Oveta Culp, 29
Hoit, Judy, 195 n. 81
Holbert, Dr. Duncan A., 162, 164
homosexuality, 102–3, 109, 113, 115–16, 127, 203 n. 113
Horizontal Man (memoir), 197 n. 141
"How America Lives" (series), 44, 46
Howe, Louis, 175
How I Became a Human Being (memoir), 76–77
Huse, Robert C., 61–62

infopolio (online discussion group), 167
In Love with the Daylight (memoir), 86
interpretive community, 138
Interrupted Melody (film), 24, 170, 172–76, 207 n. 7
In the Shadow of Polio (memoir), 72, 74–75
iron lung, 11, 12, 13–14, 16, 17, 26, 29, 32, 54, 113, 116, 118, 194 n. 64, 196 n. 127; as "iron cradle," 85; as "steel cocoon," 85

Jaffe, Rona, 112–16, 126
Jim the Boy (novel), 123–24
Justice for All, 168

Kehret, Peg, 167
Kendall, Gillian, 76
Kenny, Elizabeth, 29, 84, 171–73, 178, 207 n. 4
Khrushchev, Nikita, 80
Kingery, Kenneth, 78–80
Kinsey report, 184 n. 3
Kitsmiller, Mary, 30

Kluger, Jeffrey, 167
Köepf, Michael, 123, 125
Kriegel, Leonard J., 63, 65–67, 86, 90, 93

Ladies Home Journal, 27, 29, 34, 35, 42, 44, 184 n. 3
Land, Janet, 149
Laurie, Gini, 24, 135–37, 142, 161–62, 165, 166, 168
Lawrence, Marjorie, 24, 170, 172–75, 178, 179, 207 n. 4
Leave Her to Heaven (film), 171
Leavitt, David, 108–10
Leplin, Emmanuel, 161, 162 (fig. 6), 163 (fig. 7)
Lerman, Rhoda, 199 n. 9
Lidunska, Noreen, 71–72, 74, 75
Life, 27, 184 n. 3
Life Prints (memoir), 70–71, 110
Lightfoot, Jack, 149
Lightning in July (novel), 198 n. 7
literature-and-medicine studies 17–19, 56–59
Longest Winter, The (novel), 199 n. 14
Looking Up (memoir), 72, 73–74
Lucy (novel), 199 n. 9

Mainstream Magazine (magazine), 167
March of Dimes, 15–16, 23, 28, 29, 33, 68, 84, 97, 98, 120, 135, 153, 177, 185 nn. 8 and 14, 198 n. 8, 204 n. 9, 205 n. 26
marriage, 145, 156, 204 n. 18
Marugg, Jim, 67, 68, 76, 194 n. 64
Mason, Mary Grimley, 60, 61, 70–71, 73, 75, 86, 110, 195 n. 81
McCall's, 27, 35, 44, 45, 48, 184 n. 3
McLaughlin, Ann L., 198 n. 7
McNeill, Don, 32
Mee, Charles L., 81–85, 90–93, 197 nn. 152 and 156
Meriwether Inn, 15, 142
Milam, Lorenzo Wilson, 64, 67, 86, 88–90, 93, 183 n. 5, 197 n. 143
Mink, Rozell, 149, 150 (fig. 3)
Mix, Tom, 12
Morgan, Isabel, 29

Mouth-Voice of the Disability Nation (magazine), 167
Ms. Wheelchair America, 168
My Last Days as Roy Rogers (novel), 112, 119–22
My Place to Stand (memoir), 14, 64–65
My Polio Past (memoir), 71–72
My World Has Access Now (memoir) 195 n. 81

National Council of Catholic Women, 185 n. 8
National Council of Negro Women, 185 n. 8
National Federation of Women's clubs, 185 n. 8
National Foundation for Infantile Paralysis. *See* March of Dimes
Nazis, 99, 126
Nebraska and the Fight Against Polio (compilation), 153
Needham, Jane Boyle, 72–75
Nevis Mountain Dew (drama), 193 n. 52
Newsweek, 27, 184 n. 3
Nichols, Dudley, 170
Northwest Respiratory Center, 205 n. 34
Not Dead Yet, 168
No Time for Tears (memoir), 51–52

O'Brien, Mark, 76–77
O'Connor, Basil, 16
Office of War Information, 16
Oppenheim, Garrett, 60–61
Owen, Howard, 110

"paral" (nickname), 206 n. 42
Parker, Eleanor, 173, 207 n. 7
pathography, 191 n. 10
Patterson, James, 131, 133
Peel My Love Like an Onion (novel), 106–7
Peg Kehret's Blog (blog), 167
Pellow, John, 197 n. 141
P-Life (online discussion group), 167
People Will Always Be Kind (novel), 84, 98, 103–4, 200 n. 30
Plagemann, Bentz, 64–65, 67
"polio" (nickname), 12, 136, 206 n. 42

Polio: A Special Ride? (memoir), 194 n. 63
Polio Chronicle (newsletter), 138–41, 145, 149, 152, 166
Polio Journal (magazine), 205–6 n. 35
Polio Living (magazine). *See Accent on Living*
Poliomyelitis: definition of, 13–14; history of, 15; summertime appearance, 14, 17, 31, 36–43, 116–22; as "past," 22–23, 97–134, 198 n. 1; and the dangers of water, 35–36, 38–39, 187 n. 46, 189 n. 96
Polio Parents groups, 205 n. 28
Polio Post (newsletter), 153, 205–6 n. 35
Polio Tragedy of 1941 (memoir) 190–91, n. 7
Polio's Legacy: An Oral History (memoir), 166
Post-Polio and Independent Living Conference, 165
Post-Polio Health (newsletter), 166
post-polio syndrome, 13, 86, 98, 166, 167

race relations, 101, 120–22, 202 n. 100
Ragged Edge (magazine), 167
Rancho Los Amigos, 144, 152, 205 n. 33
Rector, Elbridge, 164
Redbook, 26, 27, 33, 35, 44, 184 n. 3
Rehabilitation Gazette (newsletter, formerly *Toomey j. Gazette*), 166
Respirator. *See* iron lung
"respo" (nickname), 160, 206 n. 42
restitution narrative, 14
Rise Up and Walk (memoir), 14, 63
Road Taken, The (novel), 112
Roosevelt, Eleanor, 173–75, 184 n. 15
Roosevelt, Franklin Delano (FDR), 15–16, 27, 70, 84, 101, 139 (fig. 1), 140, 145, 171–73, 178–79, 180, 183 n. 11, 189 n. 96, 204 n. 9
Russell, Rosalind, 171, 207 n. 7
Ryer Avenue Story, The (novel), 112

Sabin vaccine, 26
Safford, Henry, MD, 189 n. 97
Salk, Jonas, 29–30
Salk vaccine, 12, 20, 22, 26, 29, 84, 97, 107, 113, 135

Sass, Edmund J., 84, 166
Scales, William R., 157
Schary, Dore, 170
Secret Father (novel), 23, 125, 126, 128–31
sexuality, 65–68, 76–79, 105, 117, 156, 162–64, 193 n. 52
Sheed, Wilfrid, 84, 86, 98, 103
Shell, Marc, 97, 98
Sinclair, B., 148
Sister Kenny (film), 170, 172–73, 176–78
Small Steps (memoir), 167
Smith, Greg, 167
Smollar, Leo, MD, 33, 186 n. 38
Snite, Jr., Frederick, 144, 145
"Sonny's Blues" (short story), 97
SpeciaLiving (magazine). *See Accent on Living*
Splendid Solution (history), 167
Spokesman, The (newsletter), 161, 162 (fig. 6)
Stahl, John M., 171
Stalin, Josef, 128, 137–38
Stegner, Wallace, 99, 108, 110, 112, 198 n. 7
Sternberg, Dorothy, 77–78
Sternberg, Louis, 77–78, 92, 95
Strike It Rich (radio program), 45
summer camp, 30, 34
Sunrise at Campobello (film), 170–76, 207 n. 7

"This is How I Keep House" (series), 46
Tierney, Gene, 171
Time, 27, 184 n. 3
Together (newsletter), 167
Toomey j. Gazette (newsletter), 24, 135, 136, 147, 148, 153–68
Trembling Years, The (novel), 198 n. 7
Tuskegee rehabilitation center, 121, 204 n. 14
Tyndale, Bill, 148, 149, 151 (fig.4)

Uhnak, Dorothy, 112–16, 126
Van Riper, Hart, MD, 185 n. 14
Ventilator-Assisted Living (newsletter), 166
Vietnam War, 113, 193 n. 53
View from the Seesaw (memoir), 77–78

Vital Capacitator (newsletter), 205 n. 34

Walker, Turnley, 63, 67
Walters, Ann Buck, 67, 76, 194 n. 64
Warm Springs Foundation, 15, 65, 70, 84, 140, 142, 144, 145, 149, 152, 161, 164, 171, 189 n. 96, 204 n. 9, 205 n. 33
Weakly Breather, The (newsletter), 152, 205 n. 33
Wheelchair Review, The (newsletter), 145–152, 158, 205 n. 33, 205–6 n. 35
Whitelaw, Elaine, 29

Wilde, Cornel, 171
Wiley, Harvey W., 184–85 n. 7
Williams, Sue, 135–37, 142, 160, 168
"Woman and Her Car," (series), 48
"Woman and the Family Security" series, 48
World War II, 28, 29, 64, 101, 113, 126, 128, 168, 199 n. 14
Wright, Bea, 29, 68–71, 74, 75, 81–82
Wylie, Philip, 52, 184 n. 3

Yu, Jessica, 76